7/98

The Light in the Skull

The Light
in the Skull

AN ODYSSEY OF MEDICAL DISCOVERY

RONALD GLASSER, M.D.

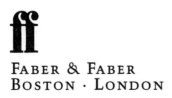

FABER & FABER
BOSTON · LONDON

Library of Congress Cataloging-in-Publication Data

Glasser, Ronald.
    The light in the skull : an odyssey of medical discovery /
Ronald Glasser.
        p.   cm.
    ISBN 0-571-19916-X (cloth)
    1. Medicine—History.   I. Title.
R149.G53   1997
610'.9—dc21   96-51607
                                                         CIP

Jacket design by Janet M. Clesse
Printed in the United States of America

*Someone very clever is going to have
to help us with this one . . .*

JOHN ROSE, M.D.
PROFESSOR OF PATHOLOGY
INFECTIOUS DISEASE CONFERENCE
AUGUST 1984

1

In the long term, we are all dead.

JOHN MAYNARD KEYNES

Despite the obvious, not all dying is the same. There are good deaths and bad deaths, deaths that are honorable and deaths to be pitied. The death of a child has little in common with the death of an adult; a soldier who throws himself on a grenade to save a comrade shares nothing with the drug addict dying of hepatitis C. Yet, in a culture in which mothers and fathers, as if no more than clouds, simply pass away, in which remembering this friend or that acquaintance is reduced to mechanics and they are merely said to have expired, all death is lost, and with that loss goes the knowledge of how to live and how to stay alive.

Perhaps there is an excuse for understanding so little of death, since only recently have we learned anything about life. It is chastening to realize that the first clear demonstration that pneumonias and abscesses, cholera and spinal meningitis, the plagues of the Middle Ages and the tuberculosis and whooping cough of our modern slums were not caused by vapors, curses, an imbalance of the humors, the interposition of the stars, a slothful life, or God's retribution occurred less than 150 years ago.

In the early nineteenth century, Agostino Bassi, after a lifetime of studying muscardine, a disease of silkworms, finally established that the disease was caused by "a living vegetative cryptogamous parasite" that had invaded the bodies of his silkworms. Sitting night after night at his workbench in the silence of his laboratory, Bassi dissected thousands of infected silkworms, seeing the same tiny parasite in each worm, coming gradually to understand the inevitable and amazing implications of his discovery. Confronted by a dozen foolish and self-serving myths and ideas of illness and disease, Bassi proved for the first time that disease was caused by one living organism invading and destroying another. There at his workbench the whole of medicine, the plagues and the pestilence, the past, present, and future slowly became clear to him.

Despite the admonition of critics and the ridicule of colleagues that he was "overstepping himself" and "making too much of his little silkworms," Bassi took the leap and asserted that disease in both plants and animals was caused by animal and vegetable parasites. Wound infections, typhus, cholera, measles, and mumps were all the same, one living thing infecting and destroying another. In 1864, attacked, ignored, and abused, Bassi wrote more in desperation than anger: "While many if not almost all eminent scientists believed and still believe that contagious materials are of a specific kind, they are actually living substances."

In truth though, Bassi was not the first to try to take disease out of the realm of speculation and the metaphysical. His idea that disease was caused by living things, in some cases too small to be seen but still able to infect other living things, was not a modern concept. It began centuries before, at a time when all illness was considered to be a malfunction of the body's four natural humors—blood, phlegm, yellow bile, and black bile. The effects of the five inertia, stars, food, mind, divine purpose, and poisons, were conjured up to explain not only disease but matters of prosperity and health. Physicians throughout the lecture halls of the greatest medical schools of Europe spent their time and energies discussing which of the precious stones—sapphires, emeralds, or pearls—had the greatest therapeutic value.

But one man, beginning to write in the year 1546, had the courage to declare that, "Infection itself is composed of minute and sensible particles and proceeds from them." Fracastorius, geographer, astronomer, poet, musician, mathematician, biologist, and physician, watched as the bubonic plague, syphilis, and smallpox ravaged the people of his age. He was an astute observer, who saw the need to free medicine from superstition and dogma, returning theory and practice to the realms of reason and observation. Fracastorius had made himself into a clinician in the true sense of that word: a physician whose only concern is the best possible care of patients. He had found that he was able to distinguish three basic forms of contagion: diseases such as leprosy that appeared to be spread by simple contact; the more pervasive and more widely distributed plagues such as typhus and cholera that seemed to be spread through human contact or contact with inanimate objects such as clothes and bed sheets; and those devastating diseases like measles and smallpox that were clearly able to be transmitted over long distances without any apparent direct or indirect contact between those with the disease and those who would become afflicted.

In a world of religious dogmas where physicians blindly followed the centuries-old rules of Aristotle and Galen, Fracastorius looked with opened eyes:

There are diseases of plants which do not contaminate animals and, vice versa, animal diseases which do not attack plants. There are other diseases restricted to man or to certain animals such as cattle and so on; certain diseases have affinity for certain individuals as they do for certain organs. If we consider these contagions in-tuitively, we shall see that the contagion of a putrefaction goes from one body to another whether adjacent or distant. [It is] these seeds [that] have the faculty of multiplying and propagating rapidly.

But in the end, as with Bassi 300 years later, the pressures of dogma, tradition, self-interest, indifference, and arrogance de-feated Fracastorius as they would defeat Bassi and almost defeat Jenner; the world continued to rely on witch-hazel nuts for fever, smelling urine for diagnosis, and bloodletting for pneumonias. In that same century, Paracelsus, a scholar and physician, wrote in defense of his own commonsense theories as well as those of Fra-castorius: "Very few physicians have exact knowledge of dis-eases and their causes, but my books are not written like those of other physicians, merely copying the ancient authorities. I have composed them on the basis of experience, which is the greatest master of everything—look, observe," he pleaded, "go back to the bedside; be suspicious of eloquence, ignore cere-mony, lecture and write in the common language, proceed from reason, and move on the learning of experience." For these words Paracelsus was accused of being a drunkard by detractors, dis-missed from university positions for not being a team player, and ignored as both a troublemaker and charlatan by his colleagues.

In truth, the battle that Fracastorius and Paracelsus fought was, tragically, the precise battle that today's infectious disease experts are having to fight in Paris, New York, London, and San Francisco.

But by the seventeenth century the power of unbiased obser-vations and the rudimentary methods of science had begun to gather enough momentum for some physicians to make rea-soned conclusions, though the majority of these early physician-scientists had to pay the price of innovation. Forty-three years after publishing his treatise on the circulation of the blood, William Harvey, still attacked and vilified by his colleagues for casting doubt on the established view of anatomy that held the liver to be the source of all blood, felt compelled to write:

> To return evil speaking for evil speaking, I hold unworthy a philosopher and searcher after truth. I believe that I shall do better and more advisedly if I meet so many indications of ill-breeding with the light of *faithful* and *conclusive observation*. It cannot be helped that dogs bark and vomit their foul stomachs or the cynic should be numbered among philosophers, but care can be taken that they do not bite or inoculate their bad humors or with their dog's truth gnaw the bones and foundations of the truth. . . . Let them go on railing I say until they are weary if not ashamed.

Harvey had fared better than the Spanish physician, Servetus, who after dissecting the body's arteries and veins, including what he called the "lesser circulations" of the capillaries, had produced a correct description of the heart as a pump in his *Christianismi restitutio*, a monograph considered so heretical by the Church that Servetus was burned at the stake and his writings destroyed.

But observation, science, and the scientific method continued to gain a foothold in the ideas of the time. Firearms had been used in small quantities in European battles as early as the 1490s, but it was only during the Italian wars of the sixteenth century that artillery was routinely used and surgeons were forced to deal with its consequences. The professors of medicine, literally sitting in their marble towers, were simply not equal to the task. They assumed, on the basis of absolutely no data, that gunshot wounds were poisoned by the gunpowder and had to be cleaned with boiling oil. Ambroise Paré, a young surgeon, accepted this belief and dutifully applied scalding hot oils directly into the wounds of the screaming soldiers. It was during the siege of Turin that the large number of injured soldiers exhausted the supply of available oil, forcing him to find other treatments to cleanse the gunshot wounds. Paré set up a battlefield experiment and, instead of using hot oils, used bland, soothing lotions to treat the wounds. "I found those to whom I applied my digestive medicine to feel little pain, and their wounds without inflammation or tumor, having rested reasonably well in the night, the others to whom was used the said boiling oil, I found feverish, with great pain and swelling about the edges of their wounds. And then I resolved with myself never to so cruelly to burne poore men wounded with gunshot—see then how I have learned to dress wounds made with gunshot; not by books." Paré was the first physician to put surgery on the correct path of critical observation and experiment, rather than simply "going by the book."

But medicine as well as surgery was turning toward observation and experimentation.

In 1642, Antony van Leeuwenhoek, living in Holland and taking advantage of the newly developed lens-making skills of his countrymen, produced a compound microscope by matching a combination of convex lenses and then used the instrument to examine a drop of well water, seeing for the first time "hundreds of little beasties" swimming in the water, all too small to be seen by the unaided human eye. A few years later another Dutchman, using a similar instrument, described in razor-thin sections of cork and wood what appeared to him to resemble the sparse, square sleeping compartments of monasteries. He named these structures "cells" because of their similarity to living quarters of the monks.

The microscope became the technical and intellectual tool that single-handedly vanquished alchemy and mysticism from medicine and gave the growing religion of science an unqualified edge in the struggle against myth and dogma. Everything and anything was examined under the microscope. In France, blood was found not to be just a fluid but to contain different types of cellular elements. In England, abscesses and pus were found to be filled with tiny organisms, while molds, spores, fungi, and single-celled protozoans were literally everywhere. Some order had to be made of this microscopic world and that took the discipline of the German character.

Robert Koch, a general practitioner in Prussia and an accomplished microscopist, set himself the task of studying a mystifying but clearly epidemic disease of hoofed animals, anthrax. Koch, like other physicians of his time, was well aware that the presence of bacteria in sick animals was a potential cause of illness, though neither he nor anyone else had any real idea how these microbes caused disease, or for that matter why they might be life-threatening in some animals and not in others.

Anthrax was epidemic in the region in which Koch practiced. The deadly, though localized, nature of this disease was obvious to everyone. Whole herds were afflicted in one pasture while in another, sometimes as near as the next farm, similar herds were spared. Koch, interested in the contagious nature of the disease, used the newest compound microscope to look at the tissues of recently afflicted animals, searching for an infecting organism. Like Bassi with his silkworms, Koch found tiny microbes, rod-shaped bacilli, growing in the autopsied animals, but he had no idea how these animals had become infected or where the rod-shaped bacteria existed before they infected the animals. There were no external sores on the diseased animals, no pustules or cuts, no blisters that would indicate a site of entry, and there were no bacteria in their mouths or throats. Yet the rod-shaped bacteria were in virtually every organ of the dead animals, including the uterus. Koch discovered that the bacteria had crossed the placenta of the pregnant animals and infected the growing fetuses, leading to the spontaneous abortions that were a hallmark of the disease. Koch was faced with two problems. The first was theoretical—even though he found bacteria in the tissues of the diseased animals, that did not of itself mean that the bacteria had caused the disease. The second was that he had to discover how the rod-shaped bacteria had entered the bodies of those animals. Koch realized that he needed a way to grow bacteria in his laboratory, methods to isolate one bacterium from another; in short, he needed means to grow bacteria in pure cultures, to study individual bacterial characteristics, and then to be able to inject pure cultures of these microorganism into animals to see if any one species of bacteria could reproduce the expected disease.

In fact, to prove that bacteria caused disease, Koch had to invent a new science, which was precisely what he did. Working alone, he devised the tedious sterile techniques that allowed him to transfer single colonies of bacteria without fear of cross contamination. He developed culture media to grow pure cultures, discovering those specific ingredients needed to keep the different strains of bacteria growing and healthy. He discovered how to heat his clear starch and sugar broths, to use closed containers, and how to sterilely transfer colonies from broth to broth. He constructed tiny glass dishes that allowed him to use a microscope and make colony counts without exposing his cultures to the open air. He began an atlas of bacteria, giving the unique physical characteristics, growth patterns, and specific nutrient requirements of each strain. Not only did Koch develop a new science, but he set the standards of scientific investigation and quality control that are still in use today.

Koch used his new techniques to prove that the bacillus he'd found in the tissues of animals with anthrax did indeed cause the disease. And while he convinced himself that the bacteria had to have traveled from animal to animal, he could find no way in which the transfer had occurred or why it only occurred in certain pastures; yet clearly, injections of the bacillus caused the disease in healthy animals. The mode of transmission eluded him, but Koch persisted and, in a series of flawless experiments, proved that at one point in the anthrax bacillus's life cycle, the bacterium undergoes an amazing and totally unexpected transformation; like a caterpillar metamorphosing into a butterfly, the bacterium suddenly alters its very structure, developing a hard outer shell, turning itself into a seemingly lifeless seed, a spore that Koch, now knowing what to look for, found to cover the grasslands on which the diseased herds would graze. Koch proved that healthy animals ingested these spores and that once inside the animal's stomach, the spores broke open, releasing the anthrax bacilli. It was the bacillus form of the microbe that then burrowed through the stomach wall, entered the animal's bloodstream, and from there was carried to all parts of the body, causing abscesses and infection, crossing the placenta of the pregnant female to infect the developing fetus. Koch's discovery of the life cycle of the anthrax bacillus was so precise and so self-evident, his techniques so flawless and reproducible, that after one rather short academic battle, his view that anthrax was indeed an infectious disease caused by the ingestion of the anthrax spores was accepted by all of medicine.

It would take another fifty years, but eventually other physicians and scientists, using the microscope and Koch's methods for isolating, culturing, and growing bacteria, would discover the cause of one disease after another. The diphtheria bacillus would be isolated from the throats of patients with diphtheria; the spirochete that causes syphilis, the bacteria of typhoid fever and cholera be found in the brains, muscles, and small and large intestines of the sick and dying. The slow-growing, oblong tuberculosis bacillus was found in the lungs of patients with chronic tuberculosis, while the gram-positive *Meningococcus* was found in the spinal fluid of patients with meningitis; chained streptococci and colony-forming staphylococci were grown from boils and abscesses. The rickettsial diseases like Rocky Mountain spotted fever, caused by tiny rickettsial organisms carried by ticks, were discovered, and eventually the intracellular pneumonialike organism that caused pneumocystis lung disease. It was microbiology that took science into the very heart of medicine.

There were others, too, clinicians rather than scientists, who tried to free the art, if not the science, of medicine from the constraints of tradition and authority. In the 1750s Auenbrugger began listening to his patients' chests instead of relying solely on a description of symptoms, discovering that those distant breath sounds were indeed distinctive and could differentiate pneumonias from asthma and emphysema from tumors and heart failure. In the nineteenth century, there began to be measurement of blood pressure, and for the first time rheumatic fever was connected to the murmurs of mitral valve disease. Physicians, dispensing with the five inertia and disruptions of the bodily humors as the cause of illnesses, were able to classify the majority of diseases into six basic and ultimately useful categories: congenital defects, metabolic disorders, infectious diseases, tumors and malignancies, vascular defects, and exposures to poisons and toxins.

But in reality, the application of observation and science to medicine and surgery offered little practical benefit other than the obvious one of not doing more harm. It was only of academic interest that jaundice was caused by greenish bile salts leaking into the bloodstream from the cells of an obstructed or cancerous liver, giving the patient's skin a yellow cast, since there was no way to treat the cancer or remove the obstruction. But still there is a virtue to knowledge and the simple chronicling of reality, if for no other reason, as facts to be used later to confirm or disprove new theories and new treatments.

In 1867, Joseph Lister, a Scottish physician, published papers and gave lectures showing that the washing of hands and cleaning of instruments with carbonic acid would significantly lower the incidence of hospital infections. Decades earlier, Charles White wrote in a paper on the management of pregnant women in lying-in hospitals that cleanliness was an absolute requirement during childbirth. At the time of White's paper, puerperal fever, from the Latin *puer*, for child, and *parere*, to bear, had become epidemic in the hospitals of Europe. In reality, puerperal fever was a streptococcal infection of the uterus, specifically of the uterine lining. It is clear today that the *Streptococcus* was introduced into the womb by the hands and unsterile instruments of the attending obstetricians who, leaving the autopsy rooms and dissection classes, came directly up to the wards to examine the patients and deliver the newborns. Once introduced into the dilated cervix or bleeding surfaces of the uterus, the contaminating bacteria quickly spread through the uterus into the bloodstream, causing terrible fevers and chills. Eventually the swarms of bacteria reached the major organs and, overwhelming the patient's defenses, caused heart and kidney failure, seizures, generalized bleeding, and within days—in some cases, hours—vascular collapse and death.

The infectious nature of puerperal fever was generally recognized. The fact that these women were healthy one day and dead the next pointed to some kind of contagion. The fact that these fevers and deaths appeared only to occur on maternity wards, as well as the fact that women admitted to the same hospital but placed on other wards, eating the same hospital food, breathing the same air, and receiving the same medications did not die or become ill was ignored by the professors of obstetrics and the hospital administrators. White's plea for simple cleanliness was ignored while all manner of other theories were offered as an explanation for this terrible harvesting of new mothers. The truth is that the self-deluding debates surrounding puerperal fever, including the theory that the disease was caused by the presence of flowers, since there were clearly more flowers in maternity areas compared to the other wards of the hospital, anticipated the discussions two hundred years later at the beginning of the AIDS epidemic when the first homosexuals and hemophiliacs began to die on the infectious disease wards of the large teaching hospitals in America and Europe. In fact, the exact same flower theory of disease was offered by a number of twentieth-century physicians who noticed that the homosexuals with pneumocystic lung infections and Kaposi's sarcomas did indeed have more flowers in their rooms than did those patients without the skin tumors and the unexplained lung infections.

But one clear-thinking nineteenth-century physician used the science that was available at the time to find the cause of puerperal fever and had he been listened to, he could have cured the world of the disease, as surely as Jenner would cure the world of smallpox.

Ignaz Philipp Semmelweis, working in the department of pathology of the great Lying-In Hospital of Vienna and well aware of what was happening on the obstetrical wards of his and the rest of Europe's major teaching hospitals, was studying the postmortem report of a young pathology assistant who had died of a hand wound received during an autopsy performed on a young mother who had recently died of puerperal fever. During the autopsy the assistant had inadvertently cut his hand with the dissecting knife and within three days he, too, was dead.

Like Bassi, Semmelweis suddenly saw, as he sat in his office examining the pathology report of his young colleague, that the microscopic descriptions of the young man's organs, the bleeding vessels, the generalized hemorrhages, and the abscesses were precisely the descriptions of the organs and tissues of women dying of puerperal fever. But what was so striking to Semmelweis was not that the pathological descriptions were identical but that they were similar even though the assistant was male and had not delivered a child. Indeed, the only injury to the young man had been a cut on the hand with the dissecting knife.

It is difficult to know the particular intuition that suddenly struck Semmelweis, what reasoning he went through, why other physicians reading that same report did not understand what he so clearly appreciated. The next morning, Semmelweis began the rounds of the hospitals of Vienna. He checked the death rates on the various obstetrical wards and indeed found what he most feared: The death rates from puerperal fever were highest in those hospitals where the physicians and medical students came onto the wards directly from the autopsy rooms where they physically handled the diseased organs of the women who had recently died of the fever.

Semmelweis went back to his own hospital and demanded that all obstetricians, most certainly those performing autopsies, wash their hands and their instruments before performing a pelvic examination or delivering a child. He was viciously attacked. The boards of obstetrics and gynecology ridiculed his concerns in the most outspoken and brutal terms. The idea of disease being introduced by the hands of caring and competent physicians was not only considered unthinkable but, worse, was ridiculous.

But Semmelweis persisted. He continued to gather data showing that in those hospitals with two obstetrical services, one run by midwives and the other by physicians, the death rate from puerperal fever was virtually zero where midwives did the examinations and deliveries, even though the entrances to the two wards were no more than feet apart. Semmelweis also showed that death rates on wards where the professors did deliveries were reaching a staggering 80 percent. But no one listened. At first, Semmelweis was merely stunned by the obstinacy of his colleagues, but as the death rates continued to increase and women in the midst of what should have been a joyous, hopeful time vomited up blood and died, Semmelweis took to stationing himself in the doorways of the obstetrical wards of his hospital, physically forcing any physician who wanted to enter to first wash his hands in a basin of diluted carbolic acid. In one of the saddest and most ironic chapters in the history of medicine, Semmelweis was driven mad as much by the screams of dying women as the refusal of his colleagues to even try to stop the epidemic by something as simple as merely washing their hands and died two years after being committed to an insane asylum, dying of a disseminated streptococcal infection caused by the ill-fitting shackles that he had been forced to wear.

It is clear today that two separate and supposedly unrelated events came together in the late eighteenth and early nineteenth century, resulting in the totally unexpected and disastrous consequences for pregnant women. In a vindication of complexity theory, where small alterations in large systems can and will lead to unexpected and unpredictable consequences, the study of pathology that had become part of the new and growing *scientific* basis of medicine suddenly combined with the emergence of the large teaching hospital to yield a quite unexpected result. The histological examination of diseased organs for educational purposes was considered to be an absolute requirement for a medical degree, while the development of large, multidisciplinary hospitals where professors of anatomy, surgery, and medicine could examine and treat patients brought to them, rather than having their own individual clinics and practices, was thought to be a considerable pedagogical improvement over the previous rather haphazard method of apprenticed medical training. In reality, though, this intermingling of disease, education, and treatment simply provided a new and deadly vector for the spread of infection—the practicing physician.

A less theoretical and decidedly more malicious view of the epidemic of puerperal fever is that when presented with the statistical facts about the spread of the disease, physicians in their arrogance and need to maintain the prestige and respect of the new, well-endowed establishment hospitals of which they were a part won out, and the women were simply left to die. It is not an unreasonable assessment. This same type of self-serving occurred in the 1980s when blood bank officials refused to admit—even to entertain the idea—that their blood supplies, particularly the pooled plasma samples being given to hemophiliacs, were contaminated with a new and dangerous virus. A less dramatic but more extensive example of such pious self-serving was the pharmaceutical industry's refusal to support or fund research that sought to prove that ulcers and stomach cancers were not caused by stress and too much acid production but by a specific type of bacterial infection.

For the past fifty years, medical textbooks and professors of medicine stated without reservation that the stomach was a sterile environment, that the high acidity of gastric secretions left the lining of the stomach free of all bacteria. The idea of the sterility of the stomach had become so much a part of medical dogma that if physicians saw or found bacteria in the stomach of a patient either during surgery or after a biopsy examination, they did something incredible—they dismissed what they saw as not being there, or more often, they asserted that what they found was contamination—which was worse than not being real—since it meant that the specimens had become infected in the laboratory during evaluation, though in truth they could not explain the path of that contamination. The weight of authority and dogma concerning a sterile stomach has been so powerful that for decades well-meaning physicians who did find bacteria in stomach samples completely refuted what they saw and did what Paracelsus and Frascatorius had warned should never be done, refused to believe their own observations.

The medical community simply decided that gastric distress and ulcers, the most common of human complaints, was of psychosomatic origin, a result of modern-day life, and psychologists and a growing number of therapists, all too willing to take over the responsibility for this common disease, put their own spin on it, writing and talking at length about our contemporary society with its "competitive strivings that trigger in people an excessive release of gastric juice that is in reality a throwback to the jungle period of man's evolutionary development." It was all very entertaining, resulting in highly lucrative profits for both the self-help industry and the drug companies pumping out their billions and billions of antacids and stress relievers.

But scientists in Australia, apparently less susceptible to the psychobabble about what is clearly a physical condition, continued to wonder about the physical nature of ulcers and continued to look. In early 1979 a pathologist at the Royal Perth Hospital examining biopsy specimens of stomach tissue found corkscrew-shaped bacteria in a few samples and refused to dismiss what he saw. He found these strangely shaped bacteria in a number of other gastric specimens and talked about his discovery with his colleagues and some of his students.

A gastroenterologist at the beginning of his career, Dr. Barry Marshall, heard the pathologist mention the strangely shaped bacteria and with what was clearly the abandon of rebellious, if unguided, youth decided to look at the gastric biopsies of his own ulcer patients. He looked closely and found at least a few of the same corkscrew-shaped bacteria in virtually all of the specimens. Marshall took the jump so common in those about to refute established tradition. He believed what he saw and decided to do the unthinkable and ignore the standard view of a sterile stomach, assuming that what he was seeing was indeed there and that the stomach, or at least parts of it, were not as sterile as everyone assumed. He continued to look at biopsy specimens, used better tissue stains, took more microscopic sections, and in early 1983, he presented his theory of a bacterial etiology for gastric ulcer disease to a group of infectious disease experts meeting in Brussels. The scientists literally laughed. The director of the Division of Infectious Diseases at the Vanderbilt School of Medicine was there that day and later admitted that the talk struck him as, "The most preposterous thing I'd ever heard."

Marshall, shaken as much by the ridicule as the criticism, was helped by a few believing colleagues. Luckily bacteriology had progressed far enough by the 1980s for Marshall to be able to isolate, culture, and grow these corkscrew-shaped bacteria which he called *Helicobacter pylori*. At first he injected pure cultures of the bacteria into rats, but nothing happened. He then fed the bacteria to baby pigs and again nothing happened. The animals did not develop ulcers and all the biopsies of gastric tissue proved negative. Apparently these animals, living as they did and eating what they did, had stomach linings resistant to the bacteria. But Marshall understood that different animal species have different susceptibilities to infections and decided to use himself.

He brewed up a pure culture of bacteria and drank it. A week later his breath became foul and he started to look pale and drawn. He developed headaches and gastric distress. Two weeks after he'd swallowed the bacteria, he had himself endoscoped by a colleague and his stomach lining biopsied. The microscopic slides showed the red, swollen gastric membranes of a shallow ulcer, and around the ulcer were swarms of *Helicobacter pylori* bacteria. Marshall published his findings in the *Medical Journal of Australia*. Many still tried to dispute his findings, but there were others who, convinced by his data, were willing to believe that ulcer disease was due to a bacterial infection. And they were right.

In 1989 the bacterium was found to be a subspecies of *Escherichia coli* that had adapted itself to the stomach linings of primates, especially humans, where it had learned to live and grow in low-oxygen conditions surrounded by a highly acid environment. The corkscrew shape had evolved to allow the bacterium to burrow into the stomach wall as an anchor to hold it in place when the stomach emptied and its contents flushed out into the small intestine. There is nobody today who doubts that *Helicobacter pylori* is the cause of ulcer disease and, in all probability, of stomach cancer. By the beginning of 1990, a hundred academic papers from a dozen different university divisions of gastroenterology had documented the elimination of recurrent ulcers in patients treated with simple, inexpensive antibiotics. The prestigious British medical journal *The Lancet* put the whole issue of ulcer disease quite clearly:

> *Helicobacter pylori* is arguably the commonest chronic bacterial infestation in man. It would have been unimaginable that such seemingly diverse diseases as gastritis, gastric ulcer, duodenal ul-

cers, and the intestinal form of carcinoma would be different manifestations of an infection with a single bacterium. The unimaginable has happened.

Marshall, continuing his studies, had become convinced that the even more common condition of indigestion, or what the internists call "nonulcer dyspepsia," is itself the result of a mild, less chronic infection with *Helicobacter pylori*. But here again, he has been challenged as having overreached himself, forcing Marshall to write what so many have written before:

> A lot of experts up in their ivory towers believe that nonulcer dyspepsia is a psychiatric or functional disorder. . . . What I see is a forty- or fifty-year-old woman with a twenty-year history of vague digestive symptoms—pain, discomfort, never gets worse, never gets better. Usually she's seen a lot of doctors, men, and they can't find anything wrong so they say she's neurotic. Usually she's had her gallbladder removed, which made no difference, probably only made things worse. I don't think these women are crazy. But it has been very difficult convincing my colleagues of that.

Medicine, whether in the past or the present, has never done well for itself or for its patients by dismissing focused observations or ignoring scientific fact . . . and nowhere has this been more obvious than in the study of infections and the relationship of infectious disease to the world of cells, cellular function, and DNA.

2

The longer he talked of honor,
the faster we counted the spoons.

WILLIAM WORDSWORTH

In the early 1980s, the World Health Organization held a little-known and not publicized conference in a small town in southern France. The conference was attended by representatives of most of the agencies of United Nations dealing with central Africa. Enough medical data had filtered out of the clinics and hospitals throughout Nigeria, Zaire, and Tanzania to force the administrators of the various international organizations to call a meeting in hopes of forming some kind of investigatory task force. The concern of the World Health Organization was not the spread of what was clearly a devastating disease but the ages and social positions of those people affected. The incidence of what at the time was called "the African wasting disease" appeared to be highest among the very people who, from a public health standpoint, should have been the healthiest, those between eighteen and forty-five years of age. It was the young, the vigorous, the military officers, the politicians, police officials, nurses, doctors, businesspeople, lawyers, judges, factory workers, truckers, and miners, those most responsible for the economic growth and political stability of their developing countries, most at the beginning of their careers, who were becoming ill and being admitted in ever-increasing numbers to the area's clinics and hospitals. The symptoms were all the same, chronic diarrhea, generalized weight loss, enlarged lymph nodes, and an increasing number of strange and virtually untreatable bacterial and fungal infections. There were also a growing number of reports concerning mental derangements, specifically short-term memory loss, and in some cases unexpected and unexplained psychosis.

The dangers of a political or military establishment in the hands of deranged elected officials or military officers were only too clear to those present at the conference. There were real, though whispered, concerns about the loss of all professional classes, the destruction of industrial bases, and the eventual failure of whole societies.

The preliminary report was considered too grim to be offered for general release. Indeed, the governments of central Africa attacked the committee's report as racially motivated, challenging the health organization's apocalyptic view of the future. Those same governments, denying that there was anything wrong, refused to allow the World Health Organization to send medical technicians into their countries to examine patients and collect blood samples. A decade later these governments would still be denying that there is a medical problem.

Yet the concerns of the task force proved to be correct. By the early 1990s, the societies of central Africa were in shambles. Their medical systems had been overwhelmed; in some areas the number of orphans outnumbered the children of intact families; economies were on the verge of collapse. In less than a decade, whole villages had simply ceased to exist, while in the cities thousands of people, unaware they were even ill, were beginning to die.

What the African politicians have forgotten, and what the

governments of Europe, America, and Asia still choose to ignore, is that survival, specifically our survival either as individuals or as a species, has never been assured or guaranteed. We
exist today as we have always existed because in the long struggle of evolution there began to develop in our ancestors, to be
passed on to each of us, a system of protection so sophisticated
and so powerful that despite a billion years of abscesses and
meningitis, burns, pneumonias, and ruptured appendices, we
have prevailed and been permitted to go on. What has been obscured and then lost is the understanding that from the very beginnings of our existence it has been those millions of unseen
microbes, the thousands of bacteria and viruses, the molds and
fungi more than any cataclysm of nature, even more than our
own foolishness and arrogance, that have been our real enemies
in the battle to survive. Our most important battles have been
waged in places so remote as to be virtually unapproachable, in
areas too small to be measured, fought with weapons we are
only now beginning to understand.

3

*Physicists make no attempt to explain why things
obey the laws of electromagneticism or of gravitation.
The law is the law and that's all there is to it.*

ROBERT WRIGHT

The science of immunology is barely a hundred years old, yet the processes it deals with are as old as the earth itself. The way our bodies fight infections began even as the earth was cooling. It has developed along with the oceans and the continents, evolving along with life itself, so that today the antibodies flooding our circulation, as well as the lymphocytes, macrophages, and neutrophils that patrol our tissues, are as real as the rocks we walk on and as fundamental as the air we breathe.

The fluids in our bodies mimic the primeval seas in which life began. The concentrations of sodium, potassium, and chloride in our bloodstreams, the calcium, magnesium, and zinc in our cells are precisely the same as those that existed in the earliest seas.

We retained those ancient seas within us, and the chemical battles fought at the beginnings of life are in reality the same battles being fought today. The battlefields may have shrunk from tidewater inlets to a few cubic centimeters of blood, from ocean fronts and shallow bays to the tissues of our brains and the plasma bathing our hearts and lungs, but failure now means the same as failure then—death and decay, the end of all that has gone before and all that might come after.

Our earth is estimated to have begun some 4 billion years ago. If there was no passion in its making, then it came about in the grim fastness of heat and fire. What gigantic catastrophe produced its beginnings, what other worlds had to be consumed, what super novas exploded, galaxies wrecked so that here in this corner of the universe a new world might be born can only be imagined. But whatever its origins, approximately 4 billion years ago here at the edge of the Milky Way in the center of a newly forming solar system spinning through a haze of galactic dust and interstellar debris, the flaming mass that would eventually become our earth began to condense and slowly cool.

What is on earth today was being molded back then; all the elements from argon to mercury, the zinc and carbon, the tons of gold and silver, the mountains of iron and lead, all the sodium, chloride, and potassium that would eventually fill the oceans and form the continents were there, superheated and uncombined, floating free in that original molten mass.

The processes that brought life about and then sustained and nourished it began as the earth, rotating slowly in the vastness of space, continued to lose heat. As temperatures dropped below 3500 degrees, chemistry took over from physics. The elements, no longer held apart by the searing temperatures of the newly forming planet, began to combine one with the other. Atoms of hydrogen and oxygen swirling in the heat came together to form great clouds of steam. Nitrogen and hydrogen combined to form ammonia; burning methane bubbling up through a shifting mantle of red-hot carbides circled the earth, forming a haze so poisonous that life was not only unimaginable but impossible. But as the denser surfaces cooled and temperatures dropped below 700 degrees, the heavier elements began to settle out into a molten core, while lighter metals rose and fell as incandescent vapors in the newly forming drifts of superheated steam. Violent electrical storms raged across the hardening crusts of future continents, while tons of molten carbon and iron spilling out of thousands of cracks and fissures boiled up into the glowing atmosphere.

All this is not mere speculation. In the early 1950s, scientists at the University of California simulated the physical conditions of that remote period of superheated steam, molten metals, and poisonous gases. Researchers filled a bell jar with an atmosphere of methane, carbon dioxide, and water vapor; they heated the mixture and then sent currents of electricity through the jar. Out of that primitive mixture came hundreds upon hundreds of complicated carbon molecules. From a bell jar containing only simple gases saturated with nothing more than heated steam came sugars and alcohols, amino acids, aldehydes, and ketones.

The importance of what later became known as the Bell Jar Experiments was not that very complicated organic molecules could be produced from simple gases but that those same molecules are today formed only during biological processes. In short, the organic compounds formed billions of years ago totally by chemical and physical processes are now the sole and exclusive province of living things, the currency of biology. Life was not only assembled from a chemical array that was, gas for gas and element for element, the atmosphere of our earth as it cooled down below the temperatures of superheated steam, but that chemistry was then taken over by life to make more of itself. It appears that as part of biological evolution, the chicken did indeed appear before the egg.

For over 100 million years the whole earth was a bell jar, a brew of steam, ammonia, heated iron and copper, methane, carbon and nitrogen compounds, aldehydes, sugars, and amino acids all adrift with one another, and not in the ounces and grams obtained in the laboratories of the University of California but in the hundreds of millions of tons. For a half-million years the earth itself formed the carbon and hydrogen-linked amino acids and circular sugars, the rectangular ketones and branch-chained fatty acids, the flat rigid carbon and nitrogen purine and pyrimidine molecules and phospholipids that would eventually become life's clay. Today's oil reserves, the billions of barrels of carbon compounds locked into the earth's crust, represent only a small fraction of the total amount of carbon-based compounds washed out of the earth's atmosphere during the prebiological age of a chemically active earth. But we now know that it was not only the earth that produced organic molecules. It was an inevitable process going on everywhere in the universe. Astronomers have shown that the hydrogen atoms in the centers of distant galaxies combine with oxygen to form molecules of water (H_2o) and with carbon and nitrogen to form clouds of ammonia and even amino acids. Asteroids captured from space have been found to contain very complicated carbon- and nitrogen-based polymers.

But here on earth, as surface temperatures cooled below 212 degrees Fahrenheit, chemistry did indeed turn into biology as water vapor held so long in the atmosphere as steam began to condense and fall as rain. Great curtains of warm rain, rising and falling, drenched the hardening earth, cleansing the atmosphere of the tons of organic compounds, carrying the sugars and ketones, the nitrogen- and carbon-based purines and pyrimidines, all the different species of alcohols and aldehydes down into the newly forming lakes and developing oceans.

There is an argument today about where these complicated carbon molecules began to accumulate. Some early scientists, including Charles Darwin, postulated that these compounds grew more concentrated in the developing coastal inlets and shallow tidewater pools. More recent investigators have suggested that life had to begin in the earth's darker, more protected places where, safe from unexpected shifts of currents and tides and the disruptive effects of ultraviolet radiation, the gathering brew of organic molecules could mingle and interact without being disturbed or destroyed. In the 1970s, geologists discovered chimneylike structures shooting up geysers of scalding hot water from hydrothermal vents along the ocean's deepest trenches. These geologists proposed that the chemistry of life was initially assembled down in the silent confines of these trenches where organic molecules, settling to the bottom of the ocean basins unaffected by changes in light or heat, water movement, or the changing tides, continued on with evolution based solely on the physical stability and intrinsic chemistry of the different molecular structures.

Twenty years ago, using remote-controlled deep-sea submersibles, scientists began to explore the seemingly hostile environments of these thermal vents and were astonished to find very primitive single-celled microorganisms living alongside the vents, surviving on bits of elemental sulfur carried up from the earth's core in the geysers of heated water. Other ancient sulfur-utilizing bacteria, similar to those found living along side the deep-sea vents, have been found in the surface baths of Yellowstone National Park's hot springs. Biochemists have calculated that at high temperatures organisms can indeed extract more energy from what are clearly calorie-poor nutrients than they can in environments of lower temperatures. Scientists using this "hot world" hypothesis of life's origins have used the discovery of these primitive sulfur-utilizing bacteria along with the biochemical calculations of energy transfers to propose that life had to be first assembled in the protected heated depths of the world's oceans.

Other theorists, focusing on time lines rather than temperatures, have postulated another scenario that, literally, reaches beyond the stars. It came as a shock to the scientific community in the early 1990s when the fossilized imprints of eleven different species of single-cell algae were identified in rocks proven to be over 3.5 billion years of age. Many of the fossils resembled present-day blue-green algae. The importance of the fossils was not only that single-cell organisms had emerged from the

primeval soup at least 2 billion years earlier than anyone had expected, within a bare 500 million years of the formation of the
earth itself, but that cellular evolution had already proceeded far
enough by then for division into subspecies to have taken place.
A number of scientists have become convinced that there was
simply not enough time in the short period between the earth's
cooling and the evolving of subspecies of blue-green algae for life
to have been assembled from all its own parts, and that life could
not have evolved on earth but was brought here embedded in asteroids coming from outer space.

The sheer power of life's chemistry became clear to everyone
with the discovery of primitive cellular structures embedded in a
meteorite torn free of Mars and thrown halfway across the solar
system to be discovered on the ice layers of Alaska. Electron
microscopy of ultrathin layers of the meteorite show the unmistakable outlines of cell membranes, while chemical analysis in-
dicates organic sugars and alcohols within and surrounding these
cell walls. The discovery of this extraterrestrial life form has
given credence to the theory that life did not evolve on earth but
was brought here through space and at an earlier time than even
the evolutionists had thought.

But where life began is less important than how it began and
how it sustains itself. Life's beginnings may be shrouded in mystery, the miraculousness of its origins obscured by theory, but
the greater mystery is not life's beginnings but its incredible
tenacity. Life's endurance, its survival, growth, and dominion—
these are qualities as rare as birth, and of these we do indeed
know a great deal.

It is now accepted by all scientists that whatever the cause
life did indeed arise in the primeval chemical soup, washed out
of the earth's early atmosphere, gradually saturating small areas
of the developing seas and oceans. The precise wizardry, whether
internal or external, that took the first of the thousands of organic molecules across the boundary from chemistry into self-

sustaining life is only now being unraveled by the new science of molecular biology. Yet it has always been clear to those thinkers who were able to not lose the forest for the trees that life, like any great enterprise, not only required a basic order and rigorous discipline to be successful but a means of taking that persistence and continuity to levels quite beyond the simple intermingling of different molecular species.

The idea of something as dynamic and dramatic as life evolving from separate inanimate molecules all coming together to finally burst forth into not only one kind of living thing but literally thousands has troubled laymen as much as it has baffled scientists and has given rise to virtually every kind of speculation. No real thinker or scientist is ever comfortable with ideas that can't be measured or concepts that defy quantification. Yet, somehow, out of that original primeval soup of disparate rainswept molecules did come a new kind of order.

For over fifty years scientists have had no choice but to take the tricky, dangerous, and at times ridiculous road of working backward from results to theories and from theories to unsupported and then insupportable ideas. In the process they have proposed all kinds of associations among the original organic molecules, clay crystals, ocean bubbles, meteorites and even aggregates of pyrites to explain how these first molecules were forced to arrange themselves into regular patterns so that physical order could be established and intimate chemical and energy interactions produced. All this speculation about a hot world or deep-space origin of life has been no more enlightening than the medieval arguments about the number of angels that could dance on the head of a pin. What biologists clearly needed were new ideas, new ways of thinking about how small things turn into big things, and how the simple becomes complicated. One critical element that had to be considered in any reasonable approach to life's evolution is that during the hundreds of millions of years when organic compounds were forming in the atmosphere and later were being washed down into the seas, the earth itself was sterile. There was no life, only a heated atmosphere of organic molecules and a cooling sphere slowly filling with warm oceans. There is no doubt that the sugars, fats, alcohols, amino acids, nitrogen- and carbon-based purines and pyrimidines washed out of the atmosphere began to accumulate and that over a long period of time it was only the most stable of these molecules that survived and finally prospered.

Molecular survival originally depended only on physical integrity. Without an atmosphere to form oxidative products or organisms to use molecules as energy sources, existence was based solely on structural soundness and chemical stability.

Those sugars, alcohols, fats, and amino acids that were the least stable slowly disintegrated, their fragments mingling with other organic debris, while the most physically and chemically stable of each class of compounds over time remained and, by default, increased in concentrations.

It was truly a Darwinian survival of the fittest. Those molecules containing the wrong combinations or arrangements of carbon and hydrogen atoms or those produced with a physically unstable three-dimensional structure gradually came apart to die and dissolve away. Under the pressures of a few more million years, even those compounds with only minor structural defects slowly began to unravel and, like their less sound brothers and sisters, started to fall apart, so that eventually only the soundest of the sugars, the most stable of purines and pyrimidines, and the strongest of the alcohols and aldehydes triumphed. Whole species of molecules, thousands of different combinations of carbon-bound sugars and scores of dissimilar amino acids must have vanished so that eventually only the six- and seven-ringed sugars, the shorter-chained fats, and the five stronger and flatter nitrogen-based adenines, guanines, cytosines, uracils, and thymidines survived, while the clumsier ten- and twelve-ringed sugars and the less fit branched-chained aldehydes simply faded away.

Recently a scientist working on the differences between molecular structures in living things decided to see if the old statistical prohibition against comparing apples and oranges applied at the molecular level. It was at best a whimsical exploration but it proved an important evolutionary concept. The scientist sectioned the two fruits and submitted dried samples to spectrographic analysis. There was no difference in the infrared spectra. The analysis proved that on the most basic molecular level the readouts of the two samples were so close that no one looking at the graphs could indeed not tell an apple from an orange. The molecules making up these two separate and apparently unique objects were exactly the same. The surfaces of living things may look different, but their internal structures are all basically the same.

The molecules that had survived the half billion years of lifeless adaptation became the basic clay of all life. What was present in the chemical soup that preceded life, those classes of molecules that because of their own internal strengths managed to continue to exist once washed out of the skies, became the building blocks of life itself. But the explanation of how the few eventually became the many had to await a new discipline. You cannot explain color if you have no understanding of pigments.

4

From so simple a beginning,
endless forms most beautiful have
been and are beginning to evolve . . .

CHARLES DARWIN

The development of chaos theory, like that of virtually any new science, began with the observations of a single man. Mitchell J. Feigenbaum, a lover of nature, simply could not bring himself to admit that the growth of clouds, the movement of ocean waves, and the paths of tornadoes were without any real or measurable order. What Feigenbaum eventually came to sense and others to understand was that tiny, almost unmeasurable variations in otherwise stable systems could, and did, give rise to totally unpredictable and unexpected consequences. Feigenbaum developed a set of mathematical rules that he felt underlay the relationships between the various levels of complexity and future outcomes, setting up enough of a theoretical outline for others to actually perform experiments to test both his theory and his equations.

The earliest and simplest experiment entailed adding grains of sand to a sand pile. Initially, adding the particles only leads to a larger pile until at some point, with the addition of a single new grain, the whole sand pile undergoes a major transformation, becoming a series of reproducible wave fronts that are both regular and symmetrical, resembling sand dunes along any shoreline. Feigenbaum's theory proposed that any simple system, when given the chance either through interactions with other simple systems or through reaching some kind of critical mass, has an inherent tendency to increase in complexity in permanent ways that cannot be predicted from the properties of any of the elements of the original systems. Even though the results of such system interactions cannot be predicted, scientists found that Feigenbaum's rules concerning what were called "phase transitions" appeared to be so general as to represent a fundamental property of any and all physical interactions. Feigenbaum's rules are used today to bring a new understanding to physical phenomena once considered to result from no more than confusion, chance, or anarchy.

In truth, the practitioners of the new science of complexity work in a twilight zone that exists somewhere between physics and computers, at the borders of order and randomness. Complexity theories deal with the evolving of phenomena within a set of predictably unpredictable parameters.

These new theorists, not as frightened of a messier and so less familiar world than the more traditional scientists, believe that all reality has a hierarchial structure, with each new level part of what has gone before but still independent of both the levels above and below. They propose that the ability of structures to change and alter peaks in a narrow range between stability and confusion and that nothing novel or unique can ever emerge from systems that have already established well-defined degrees of order.

It is this view of natural processes as part stable structure, part dynamic interaction, part phase shifts that took the study of complexity right into the center of the whole issue of the origins of life.

Computer specialists using complexity theory have produced a compelling picture of what occurred in the chemical diversity that washed into those first sterile primeval seas. Researchers at the Santa Fe Institute, a center for the study of complex systems, using computer simulations, postulated that the early chemical world was rich in such a variety of organic molecules that these compounds would eventually have formed networks, associations of different molecules that found better survival as an integrated group than as individual molecules. Computer simulations of self-sustaining chemical networks clearly give the parts of such networks an enormous evolutionary edge over any one individual component. What added credence to the survivability of such networks in the real world was the fact that the individual components in those primeval seas had already survived millions of years of molecular pruning. The networks that evolved during chemical evolution were made up of individual molecular species that had already proved their innate structural soundness and chemical sophistication.

At the time of the first publications from the Santa Fe Institute, a standard biological theory of the origin of life had won academic, if not popular, support. The argument known as the Standard Theory of Evolution presented life as a collection of simple organic molecules gradually accumulating in the world's oceans until, following some kind of random event, new classes of molecules that had the power to reproduce themselves arose.

However else biologists might view the different prerequisites for life, they understood that its fundamental quality is the ability to reproduce. They understood that early in the game the chicken did have to come before the egg and that somehow identical molecules had to learn to replicate themselves before life could take off on its own. The molecular biologists had a few of the answers, giving their own precise, if limited, structural solution to the problem of replication. It is clear that certain molecules, natural or synthetic, have a feature called complementarity: the physical ability of one molecule to fit snugly into the chemical nooks and crannies of another. The completeness of the fit depends on the different chemical bonds between the carbons, nitrogens, and oxygen atoms of the different molecules. These hydrogen-to-oxygen and carbon-to-nitrogen bonds can literally fuse two molecules together so that only enormous heat or concentrated acid solutions can separate them.

Chemists, too, have long known that the stacking of flat organic molecules, one on top of the other, flat surface to flat surface, can squeeze out any solvent between molecules, achieving a stable stacked-up configuration where each molecule survives because of the physical closeness of its neighbor.

The molecular biologists went on to speculate that eventually such self-supporting molecule structures became the dominant molecular species in the evolving chemical soup.

But the complexity theorists wouldn't buy it. First of all, replicating molecules, whatever their methods of reproduction, were— by necessity—terribly complicated structures. It was virtually incomprehensible that such intricate, yet precisely defined structures could arise by sheer happenstance in a warm pond or at the bottom of an ocean. The calculation as to the odds of a random event leading to a self-replicating molecule, much less to life itself, was too daunting for the complexity theorists to comprehend. Life is simply too complex to have resulted from nothing more than a single unexplainable random event or even a thousand such events. The spontaneous generation of life from any random event was viewed, as a recent Nobel laureate recently commented, "as unlikely to have occurred as the assembling of a complete 747 airliner by a tornado passing through a junkyard."

The researchers in Santa Fe were willing to give the proponents of the Standard Theory their primeval soup and even the billions of years of culling unstable molecules, leading eventually to a target-rich biological environment. But that was about all they were willing to give. From that point they followed what they considered to be a number of unique but scientifically sound and statistically provable assumptions. They assumed that an array of simple molecules collecting in the world's primeval soups would sooner or later undergo interactions with one another. Calculations showed that quite stable linkages between individual molecules forming chains or polymers of different lengths would result from such interactions.

Size was factored into the production of polymers. Physical structures obtain a clear biological advantage the larger and more chemically diversified they become. There has always been an advantage in nature to both size and mass. The general notion that size and complexity are not a biological advantage comes out of a distorted science fiction notion that large objects, whether giant squids or dinosaurs, because of their very size have an intrinsic predisposition to become extinct and from a less sophisticated, but more commonly held belief in this technological age, that a larger machine with more parts only means more problems. The truth is that being large gives an object or creature dimension, reducing the risks of haphazard destruction, while size and complexity allow for both a physical and chemical reach, as well as the ability to incorporate multiple and mutually beneficial functions into a single structure. In biology, structure does beget function, and the more structure, the more possible functions.

The development of a fish's fin may for generations remain no more than a means to stabilize motion, but once in place, a fin can be modified or transformed into a tail, a wing, or a hand. On the chemical level, an eight-carbon sugar might be larger and fundamentally as sound as any four-carbon sugar, but the curves and twists of the larger molecule allow for branches and connections that might be better able to protect its basic circular structure from increasing acid solutions or the disrupting effects of cosmic rays. The linking together of single amino acids to form polypeptides gives each amino acid unexpected qualities, including the ability to loop and fold in on itself, providing opportunities for three-dimensional connections as well as linkages within the polypeptide, forging a new stability combined with increasing complexity and ever newer and totally unexpected physical and chemical properties, including the ability of one polypeptide to fit in with another and then another.

The complexity theorists call these apparently small changes in systems that lead to new and unanticipated capabilities "phase shifts." Sophisticated computer simulations have shown that these phase shifts would proceed more efficiently and at decidedly lower energy levels—indeed, levels clearly available in cooling oceans—if a molecule or organic fragment were to act as a link, a physical bridge, bringing two or more dissimilar molecules together so that they might combine, interact, or feed off each other. The efficiency of the process would be greatly increased if the bridging molecule were able to unhook itself after it had brought the two molecules together and start the whole process over again. Inserting these fragments, or what chemists call "catalysts," into such computer simulations proved that by the use of catalysts whole systems could quickly be taken through a number of different phase shifts.

In 1992 a physicist, M. Mitchell Waldrop, summarized in his book *Complexity* a number of computer scenarios using small molecules acting as catalysts. The simplest and most likely evolutionary scenario was a circular one, where each component leads to its own future production. In short, a molecule A would chemically link up with a molecule B, which would then form polymer C, with C then going on to form D. With enough time and a large enough pool of molecules, structure Z would eventually be produced, closing the loop and producing more A, which would lead to more B, keeping the interconnecting cycle going, independent of any outside events. Phase shifts and self-reinforcing molecular networks all working together would under appropriate conditions eventually form a number of such self-sustaining "autocatalytic" chemical webs. It is clear from computer programs that over time the molecules and polymers of these self-replicating webs would eventually increase in concentration relative to molecules that were not parts of these webs.

But molecules within webs are certainly not life, though they exhibit aspects of being alive. There is a crude kind of reproduction here and in the simulations even a primitive competition. It is not difficult to imagine that if during a storm or tidal shift a set of self-replicating molecules were carried from one pond into another, or into a different inlet or ocean, one web might well displace a less efficient one already in place. It is also clear that different molecules and different webs, along with their own catalysts, might not only displace one another but combine and go through their own phase transitions forming new and ever more complicated structures.

But this evolutionary view in which the whole has the ability to be greater than any of its parts ignores two basic realities of existence.

The first is that during the time of chemical evolution the earth itself was undergoing its own transformation. Newly forming rivers were carrying parts of the developing continents into the seas. Lead and arsenic, cobalt and iron began to increase in the ocean waters. Gamma rays bombarded the earth's surface while acids and salts changed the very seas themselves. Temperatures continued to fall, periods of darkness came and went; and whatever physical stability and chemical efficiencies had evolved in the chemical soup no longer ensured existence. The world itself was changing.

The second is the whole issue of scarcity. As the earth's atmosphere cooled and the waters grew more inhospitable, the ability to protect what had been won, as well as the ability to adjust to scarcity, became as important as phase shifts and structural integrity.

5

*We assume that being small means being delicate;
it is a dangerous assumption.*

INFECTIOUS DISEASE CONFERENCE

Replicating molecules and autocatalytic webs, indeed any thought of evolution itself, was the farthest thing from Dr. Edward Jenner's mind in the late 1770s when he opened a small medical practice in rural England. A quiet man of modest means, he had two unique nonmedical qualities—he was curious and he listened.

It had been known from antiquity that there were some diseases which, after they had once infected a person, never afflicted that person again, that injections of small amounts of certain poisons could render a person immune from larger unexpected doses. But it was Jenner, a medical practitioner of little apparent academic talent, who literally single-handedly cleared our earth of one of the terrible scourges of mankind.

Jenner, working in the rural farmlands of England, became aware that milkmaids who had acquired cowpox, a mild, smallpoxlike disease, were spared the disfigurement of smallpox. That realization, one of the most important insights in all medicine, is described in a contemporary biography in the simplest terms:

> This event was brought about in the following manner. Jenner was pursuing his professional education in the house of his master at Sodbury. A young countrywoman came to seek advice. The subject of smallpox was mentioned in her presence. She immediately observed "I cannot take that disease for I have had cowpox." This incident riveted the attention of Jenner. It was the first time that the popular notion, which was not at all uncommon in the district, had been brought home to him with force and influence. Most happily, the impression which was then made was never effaced. Young as he was, and insufficiently acquainted with any of the laws of physiology or pathology, he delved with deep interest on the communication which had been casually made known to him by a peasant.

Jenner undertook his own scientific study of this apparent immunity in the straightforward manner of a practical man. He assumed, not unreasonably, that whatever caused cowpox and protected against smallpox lay in the pox that were the hallmark of both diseases. Jenner gathered the pus from the sore of a woman with cowpox and scratched it onto the arm of a healthy child. He watched the single pustule, the pock, develop and then, as expected with this mild disease, scab over and fall off. With what must have been great interest and perhaps even greater concern, he took the pus from an adult with smallpox and injected it into the child's skin. The child did not contract smallpox.

Jenner presented his findings to the academic medical community. But as his critics said it was only one child, and the academics of medicine refused the publication of his work. If his vaccination was so effective, how did it work? Jenner pursued his experiments and continued to successfully vaccinate more and more people; but his views on the ability of cowpox to protect against epidemics of smallpox continued to be challenged.

He refused to be silenced and independently published his own monograph on vaccination. He also went on to make additional crucial clinical observations. He noted that in those who suffered from cold sores the vaccination would not take; that it was best for these patients to wait until the cold sores were gone. It was the first time a physician had noticed that one virial infection may interfere with developing immunity to another.

While the academic medical profession continued to insist that Jenner's insight was derived from an overinterpretation of wholly inadequate data, practitioners in every country, witnessing the terrible ravages of smallpox, and being unable to save or treat these patients, listened and took up the procedure until vaccination was used worldwide.

Jenner was the first scientist to use a live virus, related to though different from the disease-causing virus, to protect against an infectious epidemic. Today the Salk and Sabin polio vaccines; measles, mumps, and German measles immunizations; chicken pox, hepatitis B and H, and flu shots are all the reflection of Jenner's enormous contribution as well as his courage to continue the work even in the face of the vilest attacks. But Jenner could never really answer his critics about the whys of protection because he never understood how his vaccination worked; he had no idea that what he had discovered had as much to do with replicating molecules and the primeval seas as it did with disfigurement and death. Nor did Jenner realize that to understand what he had accomplished, future scientists would have to go back into the very beginnings of life, to catalysts and enzymes, heredity and genes, to membranes and single-celled organisms, to how organisms defend themselves and above all else—the basic and fundamental similarities of all living things.

6

*Good pitching will always beat good hitting
and vice versa.*

CASEY STENGEL

The only reasonable explanation for the rapid appearance of different species of cellular life lies in the intricacies of complexity theory with its phase shifts and boundary conditions pushing evolution forward so that in less than half a billion years after the earth had cooled enough for chemical reactions to occur, cellular life was not only firmly established in the oceans but poised to conquer the land.

The idea of the rapid pace of biological evolution occurring in the midst of a changing earth defies the notion of life's being an exquisitely balanced affair, a clockwork mechanism made up of parts too delicate to be dissected. The idea that life is composed of individual elements too fragile to be examined, where the slightest insult will not only shatter its individual components but leave the whole process beyond any hope of recognition is no more than a self-serving view offered up by a once-clumsy science, unable until the present time to work on life's secrets without destroying the very object being pursued. Yet life, for all its purported frailness, has as both a process and a force not only survived 3.5 billion years of shifting temperatures and changing tides but has come to dominate the earth and may perhaps some day dominate our galaxy and then the universe.

It was clear to the early embryologists and later to the histologists and biochemists that for all of life's apparent diversities, all living things are based on the same internal blueprint. An elephant appears to be quite different from a flower, and yet when they are dissected, both are made up of single cells all with the same spherical shape, the same outer protective wall, the same number of inner membranes, the same internal nucleus all constructed of the same amino acids, sugars, proteins, peptides, and nucleic acids.

Nature and evolution had clearly discovered what the complexity theorists using their sophisticated computer programs had found in their own simulations, namely that it is easier to solve a number of simple problems than one big, complex one and that it is not only more efficient but also more effective to build from what is already in place than to forever be starting over and over again. It did not come as a surprise to those studying complex systems when molecular biologists reported that despite the outward diversity of living things, at the biochemical and basic structural level they were all not only surprisingly similar but in many cases identical, and that amazing as it first seemed, all living things whatever their outward differences were all constructed of a combination of the same twenty amino acids. In short, life only had twenty bricks available for construction; and that is what it used; and while a brick can be used to build a bridge, construct a castle, or raise a modern ten-story building, the basic building block, whatever the final construction, is still the single individual brick or, in the case of life, the twenty individual bricks . . . nothing more, nothing less. It appeared that these twenty amino acids were the only amino acids that survived life's primeval soup.

In truth, though, we have little physical evidence of the origins of replicating molecules and chemical webs, but what happened once single-celled organisms evolved is observably clear from fossil records. Again, there was simply not enough time from the evolution of single-celled organisms to the appearance of terribly complicated multicellular creatures for life to have continually reinvented itself. Life had to make its astonishing leaps by reshuffling the old parts already present into new structures. And at least from the study of fossils we know that is precisely what happened.

In the extreme, the scientific argument for reshuffling always goes something like this: All large, complicated creatures, whether redwoods, humans, elephants, or mice, are made up of organs, and these organs are made up of tissues, which in turn are made up of billions of individual cells. It is therefore reasonable to assume, since the same basic internal structure appears in all complicated organisms, that each creature not only evolved from original single-celled ancestors but that there had to be multicellular organisms of intermittent complexity based on this combined single-cell model where the original characteristics of single-cell function were maintained but added to as more and more single cells came together in an ever more complicated structural and biochemical mix where individual talents could be shared.

It would certainly be easier and quicker for nature to bring together single-celled structures already in existence as the building blocks for its multicellular evolution than to try to build each new species from scratch. It made no sense to spend the time and energy to build an arm or a wing when with a few phase shift readjustments of internal dynamics a remodeled fin might do just as well. Indeed, why construct a whole new lung to remove oxygen from the air when a set of gills already able to extract oxygen from seawater could easily be adapted to do the same in the air. And this is clearly what happened and continues to happen. The reorganization or "bootstrapping" of simple systems from the bottom up to form more complicated systems is clearly nature's preferred method for both survival and body building. Skeptics about bootstrapping as a method of development have only to turn on their computers and begin to surf the internet. Whatever else people may think of the World Wide Web, its true great success is as a bottom-up phenomenon where tiny individual bits of vastly diverse information, united by a few very simple, basic rules, have been welded together to form an enormously complicated monster, virtually impossible to kill, where the whole is clearly greater than any of its parts.

There is a strange contradiction here and one that separates biology from all of the other natural sciences. One of the inescapable laws of both chemistry and physics is that systems tend to degenerate over time into disorder; yet in biology, the pressure is always toward ever more elaborate and complicated systems where the newly developed whole has more potential and greater abilities to cope with both internal and external changes than any of its parts or what has gone before. The evolution of replicating polymers from simple organic molecules linking together to allow communal chemical survival is one example, and probably the first, of this bootstrapping. The second would be the production of membranes, which led ultimately to the formation of cells and the development of cellular life.

Membranes are the most efficient way of physically bringing together enormous amounts of organic molecules in incredibly small three-dimensional areas. Membranes not only offer the opportunity for greater metabolic interactions but protection for those molecules embedded in their folds. There are biologists who say that the production of membranes from single molecules was inevitable. It wasn't only the membrane's ability to bring different catalytic webs together to influence and support one other or the ability to fold over molecules to protect them from the bombardment of damaging cosmic rays or shield them from changes in the surrounding water's acidity that added a new and unexpected dimension to evolution; it was also the membrane's very two-sided nature.

The potential to form an inside and an outside, to differentiate between right and left and up and down, to be able to discriminate between what is within and what is outside, and in the process of separation, to distinguish what belongs from what doesn't, what is self from what is foreign were simply too powerful an impulse not to have evolved. The exact moment when the first membrane curved in on itself and captured a microscopic bit of those earliest seas is unknown. A shift in the tides, a sudden thermal eversion, 100 million years of membranous experimentation, and there was suddenly an inside and an outside, and in that instant life was assured a secure world in which it would always prosper.

The enormous advantage of being able to stop change clearly gave the first enclosed membranous structures an astonishing biological advantage, so much so that it appears as if all the rest of biology chose that construction as the building block for all future development. That first cell, by the simple expedient of sequestering a part of the ocean within itself, virtually ensured its enclosed molecular structures a permanence that would rival the permanence of the earth itself. Those sugars and alcohols, the polypeptides and the proteins, the five purines and pyrimidines, the whole array of phospholipids, fatty acids, ketones and aldehydes were at that moment of encirclement and with that one clear-cut, nonlinear phase transition made safe from any change in the atmosphere as well as whatever future sludge might drain off any future continents.

This is no mere speculation. Today the sodium and potassium in our bloodstreams, the concentrations of dissolved salts and the cobalt, magnesium, and calcium that are maintained in our cells are precisely the same as the concentration of those dissolved salts in the waters of the oceans existing over 3.5 billion years ago. The acids in our tissues are maintained at the pH of seawater during the Precambrian era. Indeed, for a time, all evolution might well have been called "membrane evolution." More sophisticated chemical webs and more complicated combinations of proteins with greater tensile strengths, more hydrophobic bonds, greater enzymatic properties became incorporated into these membranes to maintain a stable internal environment in what was to become a history of continuous change.

The salt concentrations of today's oceans would literally destroy any living creature if it were not for the sophisticated membrane pumps that keep the salts from entering the organism's cells. *The Rime of the Ancient Mariner* has indeed become an evolutionary truth. "Water, water everywhere. Nor any drop to drink." Without cells, life would surely have not survived the rising salt concentrations of the earth's oceans, the changing sea acidity, or the dozen different ice ages.

Once biology was safely secured within its membranes, cellular life began its own evolution. While biochemistry, unlike physics or chemistry, went in the direction of a greater complexity, such reorganization required increasing amounts of utilizable energy to maintain the ever more complicated systems, and the evolving cells began to adapt to utilizing different energy sources. Tighter webs and new catalysts pushed energy transfer reactions forward at lower and lower transfer levels. Some cells learned to use elemental sulfur as an energy source, others high-energy phosphate bonds.

For over 2 billion years cellular evolution was energy poor, making do with energy sources that were available in the oceans, plodding along with little adaptation or any real change. What is clear from the early fossil records is that once cellular life developed, a few of these early organisms evolved the ability to use sunlight as a fuel to maintain themselves and provide energy for additional development. Geologists measuring the concentration of the gas xenon in the atmosphere and calculating the present ratios of its two isotopes have estimated that 80 percent to

85 percent of the earth's atmosphere was produced in the first million years of the earth's formation and that atmosphere remained virtually unchanged until abruptly, between 2.1 and 2.3 billion years ago, the oxygen produced by newly evolved photosynthetic cells entered the atmosphere and quickly, within 300 million years, rose to present-day levels. These atmospheric studies were important for the proof they offered that once intracellular photosynthesis evolved, the growth and spread of photosynthetic cells was virtually cataclysmic. And it is clear why. The ability to use an unlimited energy source was as profound an adaptation to further evolution as was the interaction of chemical webs or the production of membranes. Photosynthetic cells quickly filled the earth or, more accurately, every place on earth touched by sunlight, and with sunlight on virtually every surface, photosynthetic cells were soon filling every sunny niche. There remained, though, the backwaters of evolution. The sulfur-utilizing bacteria living near the hot geysers along the dark ocean ridges are all that remain of the branch of cellular evolution that occurred before those same enzyme systems, feeding off energy-rich sulfides, were altered enough to learn how to utilize sunlight.

But with the proliferation of photosynthetic life, these energy-rich cells opened up a new ecological opportunity, and evolution for took a decidedly nasty turn.

It little matters to a cell's internal structures whether the cell manufactures its own energy-rich substances produced from sunlight to maintain its integrity or whether it uses the energy-rich molecules produced by another cells. In addition, there were still the nights and those ocean depths devoid of sunlight to be exploited. A high-energy cell would have a biological advantage if it did not have to stay within the bounds of sunlight in order to move, grow, or reproduce. A new evolution may very well have started with a few cells ingesting parts of other dying or disintegrating photosynthetic cells and utilizing the other cells' energy-rich compounds to feed their own enzyme systems. With the initial scavenging and the immense availability of all kinds of photosynthetic cells, the ability to use other cells' energy systems soon escalated and some lines of cells gave up photosynthesis for the pursuit of other cells. The ability to bypass the sun and utilize the energy in photosynthetic cells had the same enormous unexpected consequences that the sun had generated just a few billion years before for the descendants of the original sulfide-utilizing cells.

Virtually overnight, violence was everywhere, and for the first time death became as much a part of life as living. One type of cell developed spines to stab a neighbor, while another species evolved the ability to digest softer cells, only to be eaten in turn by a species of cell that had acquired the ability to poison. Cells able to move more quickly survived those that were slower, while slower cells developed the ability to cover themselves with mucus, becoming too slippery to be caught. Those that developed the abilities to run, hide, or fight back remained players in the new game of kill or be killed. But there were also other equally profound, fundamental internal changes going on in this new race for survival. Some cells developed the ability to produce "shock" proteins, polypeptides manufactured internally whenever the cell ran into extremes of heat or cold or changes in acidity, substances that stabilized other proteins that might otherwise unravel or come apart. In what must have been a series of quick and terrible chemical and physical exchanges, greater destructive ability gave way to greater defense, and greater defense to greater adaptability, until deflecting death became as important as being able to live. It is the same cycle that goes on today, less crudely and a bit more camouflaged, but just as devastating for the participants and just as deadly to the losers. And nowhere is this more dramatically and tragically displayed than in those children born perfectly formed in every way but without the ability of their cells to fight back.

7

To promote health, we must study disease.

PLUTARCH, A.D. 46–120

At approximately two months of age the average infant begins to experience the first of its six to eight colds a year. If the child is in day care, the number of infections goes up to twelve to fourteen upper respiratory infections, sore throats, and otitis medias over that same year. These illnesses are usually short-lived affairs—a few days of a runny nose, some coughing, a slight earache, a little diarrhea, and the child is well again.

In a few children, these upper respiratory infections persist. The child continues to cough, the fevers linger, there is restlessness and inability to sleep. The coughing and aching persist, the infection does not resolve, the runny nose does not stop. The parents may well take their child to a pediatrician or family practitioner. Antibiotics are prescribed, along with a decongestant, perhaps a chest x ray is taken, but the parents are assured that nothing is wrong. But the nose stays stuffed and, not being able to breathe, the child begins to have trouble feeding. A cold that the parents were sure would pass simply lingers. The parents may double the dose of decongestant, increase the antibiotics, perhaps try a home remedy; yet their child remains ill. The parents fight the growing suspicion that something is wrong but relax when the child appears to improve. But then the child grows ill again. The parents take their baby back to the doctor. Again the physician finds nothing unusual—congested nasal mucosa, a little fluid in the middle ear, a slight wheezing in the chest, maybe a rash, but nothing more. The doctor may change the decongestant, add an expectorant, explain the use of acetaminophen (Tylenol) or baby aspirin. He or she again explains with conviction that it is simply another cold or that the first upper respiratory infection has merely hung on a little longer than normal and that there really is nothing to worry about. The physician might even imply that the parents are being overly concerned.

But the child does not improve. Still unable to breathe properly, the child begins to lose weight and the diarrhea increases. There is a new apprehension in the child's face, a tension that doesn't disappear even when the child sleeps. The parents, unable to rest because of the fussiness, grow more and more concerned. The child looks so uncomfortable that relatives and neighbors begin to notice. The doctor is called again. But there is no real change. The physician may change the antibiotics, but nothing else.

With a few more calls and if the child's coughing grows worse, it becomes febrile, or the parents have become determined or distressed enough, the physician may take another chest x ray to placate the parents; but it is still negative, the lung fields completely clear. Once more the physician will console the parents, telling them there is nothing wrong and that eventually all will pass. The doctor believes what he or she says.

There have been approximately 100 rhinoviruses that cause flulike upper respiratory infections detected. Each virus has a different outer protein coat, different cellular attachment sites, but each has a predilection for cells of the upper respiratory tract; some attack the cells of the nose, others the cells of the inner ear, others the tissues lining the pharynx and tonsils, and a few the cells along the bronchi, but they go no deeper and, for the most part, cause only mild disease. The rhinoviruses are not as destructive as other viruses and do not cause great tissue damage. In the world of viruses, they are everywhere; but unlike the more dangerous herpes and measles viruses, even when they infect a cell, they are not very destructive. Even if an infected child cannot quite destroy these viruses, it can at least strike a balance where the child remains somewhat ill and cranky while the virus continues to exist. Still, the persistence of a viral infection in an infant, no matter how benign, is a clear warning that there is indeed something fundamentally wrong.

Within a month or two, the majority of infants with a persistent cold will become sicker. The coughing will produce more mucus. The exhausted parents, giving up on their doctor, will take the child to the emergency room. This time the chest x ray is positive and the baby is admitted for intravenous antibiotics. The morning after admission, the nurse will notice white spots in the child's mouth. The mother may well have noticed these spots herself but dismissed them as no more than congealed milk or half-eaten pieces of cereal. These spots are not food but the mold *Candida albicans*, a fungus that grows on any warm, moist surface.

By itself, the discovery of the *Candida albicans* growing in an infant's mouth, a condition popularly called "thrush," is of no concern. It is a common condition of newborns and is quickly controlled within a week or two by the infant's own immune system. If the infection becomes too severe, it can be controlled by antifungal medications until the child's own immune system comes into play to destroy the fungus once and for all. But to the horror of the parents and the confusion of the physicians, in this child the medications fail and the fungal infection continues to spread. The whitish plaques begin to grow over onto the child's lips and down its throat. The plaques begin to crack and bleed and the child, unable to eat, begins to cough up blood, and now everyone knows that something is terribly wrong.

Finally an infectious disease expert is called and after blood tests are obtained, the worst is discovered. An immunologist is consulted. An additional electrophoretic analysis of the child's blood simply confirms the infectious disease diagnosis. There is a conference, and the parents are given what was once and—still may be—a death sentence.

"Your child has a congenital defect," the immunologist explains, "or more accurately, a genetic defect. We don't know exactly where the defect lies, on which of the cell's chromosomes or what pattern or enzyme is missing, but we are sure that during fetal development one of the genes that codes for the development of our immune system, specifically for the differentiation of fetal cells into what we call the body's T and B lymphocytes, does not occur. If we are born without T and B cells or have those cells destroyed, we simply cannot produce antibodies or fight bacterial and viral infections. The reason your baby did reasonably well for the first few weeks after birth is that right before delivery the placenta allows the transfer of all the antibodies from the mother's circulation over to the baby's bloodstream. But these antibodies only last for three to six weeks and then the baby must be able to make its own antibodies, and your baby cannot do that. Everything else is fine. Heart, lungs, kidney, liver, spleen, brain, muscles, and bones, but because of that one genetic defect, there is no immune system; no way for your child to fight infections."

"And what can we expect?" the parents ask.

The doctor hesitates.

"There is a treatment that may help, a bone marrow transplant, where we replace the genetically deficient immune cells, but it is terribly risky . . . as many die from the procedure as survive; and of the survivors, less than 25 percent will have a good result."

"And if we don't try . . . ?"

"Your child will eventually die of a pneumonia, meningitis, or sepsis."

"And antibiotics?"

"They work, but only if the microorganism is a sensitive strain; antibiotics will keep your child alive, but only for a while. Sooner or later there will be an infection with an organism resistant to all antibiotics. We can also give monthly infusions of gamma globulin, which will contain some antibodies, but there is nothing we can do for viral infections; and eventually there will be an infection we cannot treat."

The parents are silent. There is nothing more to ask and nothing more to be said. The answer to their child's disease lies both in the past and the future, in the dissection of 3.5 billion years of defense, in understanding the ways in which tissues divide and grow, and more importantly, in how single cells talk to each other and in the midst of infections decide what belongs and what doesn't.

It was growing clear to the infectious disease specialists and the immunologist called on to care for these immunologically deficient infants that the answer, indeed the cure to their disease lay somewhere in the whole issue of inheritance, in understanding the past and bringing it into the present and then forward into the future.

8

It is like a dog walking on his hind legs;
it is not that he does it well,
but that he can do it at all.

SAMUEL JOHNSON

It has been known since the time of the Greeks that the physical traits of plants and animals as well as certain human characteristics such as height, eye color, size, and hair texture are passed from parents to offspring. But it took controlled breeding before anyone was able to see that there was a certain rigid order to this transmission of physical characteristics.

The scientific study of inheritance began in the 1860s when an Austrian monk and gardener, Gregor Mendel, saw what others had only noticed and decided to try to sort things out. There were at the time two types of cultivated legumes; one plant produced wrinkled yellow peas and the other a smooth pea with a green skin. When these different plants were cross-pollinated, the two physical traits of pea color and skin type passed on to the next generation, but not equally, at least not in the first generation. Growers understood that whatever they planted, the first generation of plants always produced smooth green peas.

But after that, the whole issue of inheritance became a jumble, and in the next generations wrinkled green peas and smooth yellow peas started showing up, seemingly out of nowhere and in unexplained proportions. Mendel decided to study this transmission of traits by carefully cataloging which plants and which offspring were pollinated, and then he used his data to repollinate during a series of extensive inbreedings, proving in the process that there was nothing chaotic about inheritance and that indeed the two physical characteristics of skin texture and color were transmitted from generation to generation in a regular and reproducible fashion.

Mendel proved that the transmission of physical traits, sometimes hidden and at other times observable, did not in any way alter or change that characteristic. After a hundred generations, a yellow wrinkled pea was still a yellow wrinkled pea, and a smooth green pea was still a smooth green pea. Two fundamental biological observations came out of Mendel's experiments. The first was strictly mathematical: specifically, that the percentages in each generation of the four combinations, yellow wrinkled, green smooth, yellow smooth, and green wrinkled, could only be explained if each trait was under the control of two different factors: one factor from each of the two original plants. The second conclusion, the one that surprised Mendel and for which he had no explanation, was that each trait appeared able to hide itself during any one interbreeding, only to reappear full-blown and unchanged in later generations. Mendel clearly had no idea what was being transferred from plant to plant or how the green color and smooth texture had disappeared in one generation, only to be completely resurrected in the next; yet he understood that what was transferred was not only permanent and indivisible but a real physical substance obeying mathematical laws. Reluctantly, Mendel took an enormous leap and proposed that all inheritance is transferred through generations as uniquely stable individual and unchangeable factors. He called these factors of heredity "genes." What Mendel didn't say was that whatever these genes were, they obviously had to be packaged within the individual microscopic pollen grains that he used to fertilize his separate plants. While Mendel was doing his cross-fertilization experiments, other scientists were convincing themselves that what worked in plants also occurred in animals and that heredity, whatever else it might be, was passed on from generation to generation as discrete units but that in animals these factors were contained within the egg cells of the female's reproductive system and the individual sperm produced by the male testis.

In a classic experiment that today seems naive but at the time shocked the established medical and religious community, an Italian biologist, Lazaro Spallanzani, put diapers on male frogs, keeping any released sperm from contact with the female's eggs. The biologist proved that if the sperm cells were not allowed to physically mingle with eggs, no tadpoles emerged. Yet when the sperm were removed from the diapers and placed on those same eggs, fertilization occurred and new tadpoles developed. It was not lost on Spallanzani or his detractors that the tadpoles that were produced from mixing eggs and sperm were not just any old tadpoles but tadpoles whose characteristics were a mixture of the physical traits from whatever species' eggs and sperm were used in the experiments. The discovery of the microscope finally proved that eggs and sperm were cells and that the *units* of heredity, or genes, had to lie in what the first microscopists called the cell's "nucleus."

The early microscopists had quickly discovered that all cells had a similar structure; there was an outer membrane, or wall, containing a freely movable viscous fluid called the "cytoplasm," from the Latin words *cyto*, for "cell," and *plasma*, for "fluid." There were numerous small granules and particles floating in the cytoplasm and a larger circular structure in the center of the cytoplasm that they named the *nucleus*, from the Latin word for "kernel," because of its central location within each and every cell. There truly appeared to be no exceptions. Sections of tree trunks, leaves, parts of fish and worms, hearts and lungs, slides made from the petals of flowers and the inside of blood vessels, every living thing examined under the microscope was composed of cells, all having the same structure and internal composition. Indeed, the new science of microbiology declared all life at its most basic level to be composed of single, individual cells. But that observation proved to be not quite correct; and indeed, a refinement of the very instrument that had once been used to proclaim the cellular basis of life was later used to undermine the same theory.

For over 200 years, biologists used the light microscope to support this view of a cellular basis of life. Embryologists observing the fertilization of different species watched the sperm cell's membranes merge with the egg's outer membrane; the two separate nuclei drew toward one another until they, too, physically joined, the two cells sharing everything, suddenly and miraculously becoming one single cell. One can only imagine the amazement as those first microscopists watched as the newly merged cell started to split down its center, one cell becoming two and the two cells becoming four, the four quickly twisting into eight, the eight becoming sixteen, and then thirty-two, until eventually a round mass of apparently identical cells began to elongate and take on the shape of the earliest fish. The microbiologists dutifully reported that the egg cell of a species was always considerably larger than the sperm cell. It seemed an important distinction to scientists looking for anything to help explain what they were watching unfold right before their eyes. A closer examination, however, showed that the size difference was due solely to the amount of cytoplasm present, the sperm having only a tiny rim of cytoplasm around its nucleus, while the egg cell, fat and round, contained so much cytoplasm that it seemed to be close to bursting. Except for this difference in the amounts of cytoplasm, the egg and sperm cells appeared to be identical, including the same centrally placed, virtually identically sized nucleus. It occurred to these first embryologists that whatever controlled a new individual's development probably lay in the nucleus rather than the cytoplasm.

A single experiment proved the point. Embryologists damaged the cytoplasm and then the nuclei of comparable eggs and sperm and found when the nucleus of either an egg or the sperm was destroyed, no new offspring developed from the merging of cells, but damaged cytoplasm still led to at least the beginnings of a new individual. The embryologists concluded that the units of heredity clearly resided in a cell's nucleus. The development of the organic dye industry in the middle of the nineteenth century began to unravel the *where* in the nuclei if not yet the *what*.

In the 1870s, German biologists were for the first time able to use the products of a developing German chemical industry to produce dyes that stained specific organic molecules. Some dyes only stained substances that contained sugars, others only nitrogen-containing molecules, and still others only alcohols. These dyes were quickly used by biologists and chemists as probes to identify different classes of organic compounds. When these different dyes were applied in a systematic way to microscopic samples of living tissues, it was found that the nuclei of cells were not simply fluid-filled sacks but contained, tiny discrete structures curled up inside the nuclear membranes that stained so darkly with a unique organic acid dye that the biologists called these structures "chromosomes" from the Greek word for "color." Surprisingly, the scientists found the number of chromosomes in the nuclei of cells to differ depending on the species and, more surprisingly, that the number of chromosomes were always the same in all the cells of any individual from any one species. Embryologists using this new dye went back to their microscopes and relooked at the whole process of fertilization. They soon discovered that at fertilization the chromosomes from the nucleus of the egg and the sperm took up a central position in the newly merged nucleus. During division of the fertilized egg, the two sets of chromosomes began splitting down their middle, the two halves starting to physically move apart as the cell itself started to divide. It was clear under the microscope that the cytoplasm of the newly fertilized cell began to pinch down between the retreating lines of split chromosomes until the pinched ends of cytoplasm finally met, joining together to form two completely new cells, each with a new nucleus containing half of the original complement of merged chromosomes.

At the time of these experiments, the organic dyes used in the original microscopic evaluations were discovered to stain a specific class of organic compounds named *nucleic acids*, polymers made up of different segments called "nucleotides." Each nucleotide consisted of a sugar molecule connected to a nitrogen-containing purine or pyrimidine molecule. Nucleic acids were in reality long strands of thousands of nucleotides all linked together.

Biologists used the discovery that chromosomes contained nucleic acids in a number of experiments known as Poison Experiments. They were sure they had the *where*, of heredity and even if they didn't know the *how* they wanted to find out about the *what*. The scientists exposed embryos to specific frequencies of ionizing radiation known to damage only nucleic acids. They found that large doses simply killed the developing embryo, but smaller exposures to a recently fertilized egg or larger exposures later in fetal development did not kill the embryo or halt embryonic growth but led instead to severe, in many cases life-threatening, malformations. Even more worrisome, these early radiation experiments proved that if the cells of an embryo were exposed to ionizing radiation toward the very end of fetal development, the results would not be congenital malformations but tumors and early malignancies. Clearly, specific damage to a cell's nucleic acids not only interfered with normal development but could lead to cell death as well as cellular dysfunction.

But there were other things about chromosomes almost as troubling as the enormous changes caused by even the slightest damage. No one could explain how a chromosome could split in half and reappear intact in each new cell. Every time a fertilized egg split, half of its chromosomes would move into each new cell, yet at the end of each division the same original number would always appear in the new cell's nucleus, no matter how many divisions of the original cell. How could chromosomes halve themselves with each cellular division only to appear whole again before the next division?

The mystery only deepened when scientists were finally able to physically extract the chromosomes from a cell's nucleus and made the discovery that whatever the species, whether plant or animal, bacterium or human, the nucleic acids making up the chromosomes were identical; they were all constructed of the same deoxyribonucleic acid, or DNA. Despite the apparent diversity of all living things, all extracted DNA appeared to be identical. Both mysteries had to be solved before anyone would be able to explain what a gene was and how it worked.

9

Irish poets learn your trade,
sing whatever is well made.

JOHN KEATS

In early 1978 a gastroenterologist working at a Zaire hospital noted a dramatic increase in the incidence of patients diagnosed with severe fungal infections, particularly the fungus *Candida albicans* of the throat, mouth, and posterior pharynx. The gastroenterologist, ignoring or unaware of the data in the pediatric literature concerning thrush infections in children born without an immune system, published his finding in the British medical journal *The Lancet* offering no explanation except the obvious, "Such fungal infections are usually seen only in those patients on chemotherapy for cancer treatment."

At the same time that the article was published, other doctors throughout central Africa were noticing a change in the patient population being seen with severe diarrhea, chronic weight loss, and severe skin infections. Patients with these constellations of symptoms had traditionally been the very young or the very old. These same patients were also found to have swollen lymph nodes, many had suffered recurrent pneumonias, some even presented with recurrent episodes of virial meningitis, and virtually all suffered from gastrointestinal parasites.

At the same time that the African physicians were discovering this new population of chronically ill patients, the Centers for Disease Control in America, the Pasteur Institute in France, and the Institute for Tropical Medicine in England were obtaining strange reports of Haitian immigrants being admitted to hospitals in their countries with diagnoses of disseminated fungal infections and pneumocystis pneumonias. A tenuous connection between the medical experience in Africa and the illness among Haitians was offered by a British researcher writing, again, in *The Lancet*, "While numerical data are lacking, it is clear that several thousand professional people went from Haiti to Zaire between the early 1960s and 1970s. Discussions with Haitians remaining in Zaire show most of these people have left to live in Europe and North America."

In truth, the Africans and the Haitians were only the overtures in what was to eventually become a terrible world-wide symphony. The tune would soon become all too evident, but at the time of those first few articles in *The Lancet* there was only indifference and confusion. In a very real way, medical science had grown too specific to see the forest for the trees. Those scientists who would prove most helpful in unraveling this new mystery would be the complexity theorists and the world's virologists, the very scientists considered to be the most misguided, because they dealt with systems.

Stuart Kaufman, one of the earliest proponents of autocatalytic chemical webs as a prerequisite for the evolving of life, put the issue quite clearly as early as 1960 when he wrote:

> The people doing the most in biology are the lowest of the low. It is, of course, exactly the opposite in chemistry and physics. . . . There is a remarkable certainty among [some] molecular biologists that all

answers will be found by understanding specific molecules . . . but there is a great reluctance to study how a system works.

Systems analysis in biology has always been considered too speculative to be of any real value, despite the participation of some of the world's greatest thinkers, including John von Neumann, who, along with Einstein, is considered to be the greatest mathematician of the twentieth century. As early as the 1940s von Neumann had developed and then constructed the first computer but soon, through his equations governing computer processing, became interested in self-replicating machines. Taking a cue from evolution, he imagined a machine constructed on a primeval pond that, instead of being filled with sugars and aldehydes, polypeptides and proteins, was filled with an infinite variety of different machine parts. He designated his machine the "universal constructor." Given any blueprint it would move around the pond until it found all the parts described on the blueprint and then, putting the parts together in the prescribed order, build the machine. Von Neumann then assumed that the blueprint under construction was the plan for the original universal constructor and that after the machine constructed its own exact replica, it would go on to produce as many of these as there were parts available.

But von Neumann realized that while all this construction looked like self-reproduction, in reality it wasn't. An important quality was missing, namely, the ability of each new machine to go on and make an additional copy of itself. If each newly constructed machine did not contain its own copy of the original blueprint, the production of all the replicas would end with only a first generation of identical machines.

Von Neumann was forced to postulate that in order for his universal constructor to endlessly reproduce itself, providing enough parts were available, the description of its own construction also had to be reproduced and those precise instructions passed on to become part of each newly constructed machine. In short, any self-replicating system needed a method to pass on the instructions for assembling its different pieces out into future generations as much as it needed the raw materials for its physical construction. A simpler biological version of von Neumann's cataclysm for self-replication states that genetic material must play two roles; it has to serve as a program to be used for the construction of an offspring while at the same time serving as a method of passive data transfer of a description of itself to be incorporated into each cell of that same new member.

But biologists paid no attention to von Neumann, despite the fact that in the 1950s Swedish chemists, working with the first truly pure samples of DNA, found that the original description of all DNA as being the same was not correct. The nucleic acids extracted from the chromosomes of cells from different species were indeed all composed of the deoxyribose sugars, but the nitrogen components of each individual nucleotide, the carbon-nitrogen-containing purine and pyrimidine molecules, were not identical. Purines and pyrimidines are very basic and very old carbon- and nitrogen-containing substances with a number of unique qualities. They are flat, platelike molecules, resistant to being bent or flexed, with high melting points and virtually complete resistance to changes in acidity, oxygen saturations, and exposure to shifts of electrolyte concentrations. In addition, these purines and pyrimidines, unlike other carbon compounds, have a unique three-dimensional construction that allows the edges of a purine to form very strong and very stable hydrogen-oxygen bonds with any other pyrimidine. As far as organic chemists have been able to determine, only four purine and pyrimidine molecules survived the primeval soup to become part of life's clay: two smaller purines, adenine and guanine, and two larger pyrimidines, cytosine and thymine.

Until the Swedes started their detailed analytic studies, all that was known about DNA was that it was a nucleic acid made up of sequences of individual nucleotides linked together and that each nucleotide consisted of the same six-carbon deoxy-ribose sugar, a phosphate molecule, and a single purine or pyrimi-dine connected to the sugar, most likely, through a common con-nection with the phosphate. At the time the different possible combinations of the purine and pyrimidine bases were considered of no greater consequence than the sugar or the phosphates. The continuing analysis of DNA showed that the percentage of the four purine and pyrimidine bases—adenine, guanine, cytosine, and thymine—appeared to remain constant in the cells of any one species, though those percentages varied greatly from species to species. Reluctantly the Swedes came to the conclusion that it was the different percentages of the purines and pyrimidines in DNA that appeared to control and define life and were, in reality, Mendel's genes.

No one believed them or, more accurately, wanted to believe. But the Swedes stuck to their interpretation and they had a com-pelling argument. DNA clearly carried the genetic code; the basic composition of DNA was understood, and on the chemical level it was quite simple. All DNA was composed of the same sugar, the same phosphate atoms, and four different combinations of ni-trogen and carbon bases. It did not take a genius to realize that since the DNA from all species contained precisely the same sugar and exactly the same phosphate molecules, and since every species differed in outward form and function, the blueprint con-trolling these differences had, by exclusion, to lie in some kind of difference in the purines and pyrimidines that made up the indi-vidual nucleotides. In short, the differing proportions of the four bases—adenine, guanine, cytosine, and thymine—making up each individual nucleotide had to be the genetic code.

Still, it was simply too fantastic an idea to entertain, much less believe, that the units of heredity held within the DNA of a cell's chromosomes were nothing more than the differing amounts of adenine and guanine, cytosine and thymine making up the strands of DNA. But there is an imperative to good science. Observations may be pushed aside, but they cannot be ignored. Galileo did indeed see the moons of Jupiter in their own specific orbits; and the cardinals of the Church, to their own detriment, refused to look and in dismissing Galileo's observations embarrassed not only themselves but also the Church. So much so that, in 1996, Pope John Paul II felt obliged to declare that the Church had indeed erred in condemning this first astronomer.

A number of scientists accepted the Swedish observations and, combining the bootstrap theory of evolution, chaos theory, and the input of geneticists, decided to keep their eyes on the prize—the individual nucleotides making up the strands of DNA—and using ever-newer technologies, continued with their pursuit of the genetic code. These DNA hunters turned to the new science of crystallography, an esoteric branch of physical chemistry using x rays to define the structure of complex organic materials, to keep them on the right path. In examining strands of DNA, crystallographers found that the width of a strand of extracted DNA was precisely the width of two nucleotides set side by side. Additional crystal diffraction studies supported these dimension studies, indicating that a molecule of DNA was not, as expected, a single strand of linked nucleotides but rather was made up of two strands, each strand somehow linked or connected to the other in a kind of side-to-side configuration.

It was obvious to a few brash young researchers that the holy grail of biology, the *genetic code,* was to be found somewhere in unraveling the riddle of exactly how this double-stranded molecule, composed of linked nucleotides that had survived the primeval soup to become sequestered within the nucleus of every cell, had originally been constructed.

James Watson and Francis Crick, two Cambridge biologists, neither older than thirty, had set themselves the task of discovering this internal structure of DNA. They had virtually no academic credentials for what they were trying to do, but like Jenner they were astute observers, and they listened and they read. They also had available to them the molecular dimensions of DNA and they knew that all DNA was composed of two nucleotide strands. There were also those data showing that the percentages of the four different bases varied from species to species. Watson and Crick, in an unconventional approach, constructed three-dimensional models of the different components of a nucleotide—the circular deoxyribose sugars, the four different, rigid, flat platelike purines and pyrimidines, and the spherical, hinged phosphate molecule, all made to precise atomic scale—and simply tried to put the different parts together. The two biologists turned themselves into model builders, trying to connect the different components of DNA in a way that made both structural and biological sense. They held the different parts of the model together with rods and clamps, twisting and turning the two unwieldy strands of nucleotides around in an effort to make the parts fit together. But no matter how they moved the parts or in what combinations, the whole thing always came out looking like some kind of crazy Erector set.

For well over a year the two tried every possible combination, but despite their best efforts nothing fit and they were left with an ever-changing unbalanced three-dimensional jumble of circular sugars and round phosphates and four different flat purines and pyrimidines. Watson and Crick knew they had all the pieces, but they could not make all the pieces fit together.

Meanwhile, the crystallographers continued their high-energy x-ray analysis, showing not only that a molecule of DNA was composed of two chains of nucleotides lying side by side but that there was a periodicity to the structure, a kind of twisting of the two strands spaced out at well-defined, regular intervals. Watson and Crick examined these new evaluations and convinced themselves that the newer, more precise diffraction patterns meant that there had to be a basic rigid backbone structure to DNA and that somehow this backbone curved around on itself in a regular periodic fashion. There was no doubt from the bonding data that the sugars of each individual nucleotide had to make up the backbones of the two strands and that the round phosphates had to act as the hinge points between both the flat bases, the sugars and the separate nucleotides, allowing the whole structure to twist through a 120-degree arc in any horizontal plane. The problems were the individual purines and pyrimidines sticking out from each nucleotide and how these bases fit into this new backbone scheme of things. But even as they refined their model, pushing the two nucleotide strands together, the flat bases sticking out in all directions from each nucleotide strand only made the combined model look more and more like a bizarre semaphore than some kind of master code.

It wasn't only their inability to figure out what to do with the adenines and guanines, cytosines and thymines that so troubled Watson and Crick; it was the overall sloppiness of their different models. They understood better than anyone that whatever the ultimate structure of DNA, even with its separate parts and different linkages, it had to be a physically stable structure that somehow still retained within itself the chemical and biological flexibility that would allow it to reproduce itself as well as direct the course of all evolution. Nature would simply not allow the survivor of over half a billion years of chemical evolution to be the least bit unbalanced or structurally unsound.

The crystallographers, though, had continued their work. At a conference in Denmark, Watson and Crick saw the most recent x-ray diffraction patterns and, in consulting with the crystallographers at Cambridge, realized that the periodicity of the DNA molecules seemed to indicate that the sugar spines of each nucleotide strand did not meet in the center of a molecule of DNA, the accepted backbone scenario, but rather seemed to run along the *outside* of the DNA. The two young men finally understood, and in less than a week they had the answer. Following the atomic dimensions of the diffraction patterns, they simply moved their model of DNA apart so that the two strands of nucleotides gave the proper internal dimensions, placed the sugar from each opposing nucleotide strand along the outside of the model, swung the bases of each individual nucleotide inward toward the center of the two columns of sugars, and watched as miraculously the whole thing suddenly came together. With simple readjustment of the distances between the two columns of nucleotides so that the bases, now in the center of the model, barely touched, the structure became a spiral staircase, the outer railings of the staircase made up of the strands of linked sugars, each of the individual steps of the staircase formed by the flat base from one railing connecting to the base of the nucleotide directly opposite—the whole twisting staircase suddenly taking on the unmistakable aspect of a solidly built, well-constructed, double helix.

In their book describing the discovery of the structure of DNA, Watson and Crick explained that they stood amazed, looking in awe at a model suddenly so elegant and so solid, where literally a few minutes before there had been only confrontation and molecular confusion. Mathematicians versed in solid state geometry were quick to point out that a double-helical structure is the most efficient form for incorporating the greatest number of structures—the complexity theorist would say "information"—within a limited amount of three-dimensional space.

However, a closer inspection of the Watson and Crick model showed some minor but substantial defects. The steps formed by some of the bases from opposite sugars either overlapped or didn't quite reach the base coming from the other side. In short, a few of the individual steps were not well constructed, forming obvious weak points in the internal structure. But Watson remembered one of the established but disregarded facts about DNA, namely, that the percentage of bases was always the same in the cells of the tissues for any one particular species but different from the DNA of any other species. Watson was also aware that the more complicated a species, the more chromosomes in the cell and the more DNA. Somehow amounts and percentages of the different bases had to be important.

Watson and Crick began to shift around the different nucleotides, changing the bases that were opposite each other, and
they quickly found that the best match, indeed, the only perfect
match, was always an adenine opposite a cytosine and a thymine
opposite a guanine. It didn't matter which strand was which; the
readjustments and substitutions finally made everything fit, the
model becoming complete when a smaller purine was always opposite its complementary pyrimidine; and in this perfect complementarity where an adenine was always opposite a cytosine
and a thymine always opposite a guanine, Watson and Crick saw
precisely what von Neumann had predicted to be an absolute requirement for any self-replicating system. The internal structure
of their double helix, the bases of the nucleotides from one railing of the ladder, were a perfect complementary image of the
bases of the nucleotides from the other side. If the helix of their
model was opened, in a way unzipped along the center connections between the bases, each complete strand would be an exact
complementary replica of the other, an adenine of either strand
always opposite a cytosine of the other and a thymine always opposite from a guanine. Watson and Crick published the structure
of DNA in the March 1953 issue of *Nature* and every scientist
and researcher in the world quickly saw what Watson and Crick
had seen, that by opening the double helix down its center, two
exact replicas of the original double polymer of DNA could be
constructed from each individual strand. The adenine of one
opened strand recombining with a cytosine, a cytosine of the opposite strand connecting to a new adenine and in that process
forming an exact duplicate of the original double helix.

Here in this simple but elegant structure composed of single
nucleotides linked through their sugars and only four carbon-
nitrogen bases was not only the means for an endless future of
molecular replication but the ability to transfer information easily and reliably, not only from helix to helix but generation to
generation.

10

If it sounds good, it is good.

DUKE ELLINGTON

There is an axiom among fighter pilots that a plane that looks as if it can fly is the one that will perform. The F-16 Falcons and the F-15 and F-18 attack bombers, so successful against the MiGs and French Mirages, all have that quality of looking right. Indeed, it is that gut feeling about visual correctness that has become the metaphysical equivalent of "form begets function." It was obvious to everyone who looked at Watson's and Crick's model of DNA, with its simple but intricate construction, that here was a polymer that simply looked the part, not only as the survivor through 3.5 billion years of evolution but as the self-replication code capable of fueling all of life's diversity. There were no scientists or researchers seeing that model who did not realize that somewhere in that model lay the answers to their own questions.

Cellular biologists saw in the two-part complementary construction the explanation of how a chromosome could be halved with each cellular division only to reappear undiminished in the next generation of cells. The DNA could split itself down its center at the beginning of each cellular division, each half of the double helix going into each new cell, only to have the polymer reassembled again; each half hooking up with its complementary nucleotides so that the two pieces, safely tucked away within the nucleus of each of the new daughter cells, would become an exact replica of the original strands of DNA.

Geneticists saw in the different array of bases the cause of mutations and congenital defects. An error in replication, an adenine somehow inserted in the place of a cytosine, and the information carried in the base sequences would be changed and that change carried forward into all additional cellular divisions. Precise self-replication was clearly so critical a part of life's stability and endurance that early in the development of cellular evolution nature placed such a priority on the exactness of DNA duplication that it evolved a backup system—beyond the formidable internal dimensional constraints of each base having to match up physically with its correct opposite—within the nucleus to check any newly constructed strand of DNA for errors of replication. Molecular biologists at Johns Hopkins University studying genetic instability in certain species of yeast discovered a small enzyme that actually travels down a column of newly forming DNA scanning the base linkages, and at any place where there is a bulge in the helix or some other evidence of an improper fit, this protein excises the wrongly placed nucleotides and directs the placement of the proper base pairs. The discovery of a "check spelling" protein that eliminates errors of replication might have been no more than a curiosity had that exact same enzyme not been found in the nucleus of every human cell. The implications are astonishing. Very early in cellular evolution a gene developed in the genetic code that produced a nuclease, a protein enzyme in the nucleus that gave that cell such an evolutionary edge in biological stability, and ultimately in existence, that the early check spelling gene was carried forward into the genetic pool of virtually every future living thing.

Scientists interested in reproduction saw in the model the reason for two sexes. It was obvious to the majority of biologists that asexual reproduction, or one individual simply dividing and making more of itself, is a much more efficient method of procreation than sexual reproduction. There is no need to find a partner, no wasted time, no risk of being attacked and damaged or destroyed while searching out an acceptable mate, and certainly no need to squander valuable energy in all the *Sturm und Drang* of a sexual pursuit. But sexual reproduction has clearly won out as nature's most successful and indeed virtually universal form of reproduction. The answer lies in the extraordinarily stable structure of DNA and what game theorists call the "lottery scenario."

What is the best way to win a game of chance? Bet all you have on one number or split your bet and place a little here and a little there? Asexual reproduction, one organism reproducing itself in perpetuity, is in reality the bet-it-all-on-the-one-roll-of-the-dice plan. If you win, you win big; but in a real world of change and probability, shifting tides, fluctuating temperatures, increasing oxygen saturations and, of course, competition, the chance of winning on one of anything grows increasingly small. Sexual reproduction allows for hedging the bet; each partner brings its own stable set of DNA to the table and in the intermingling of the two sets of chromosomes new combinations of genes, in essence a reshuffling of the units of heredity, occurs and the new genetic combinations give each new creature a slightly different ability to change, to alter itself, to be better able to cope with whatever may suddenly or unexpectedly appear.

The early oncologists saw in the model of DNA not stability but the reason for tumors and malignancies. If an error in DNA construction did indeed occur during replication, if the check-spelling protein malfunctioned or the DNA became so injured or damaged that a wrong base was inserted, a new sequence of bases and, therefore, a new or confusing blueprint would be put into operation and in the confusion lead to abnormal cellular function and perhaps even uncontrolled tissue growth. This view of abnormal or distorted growth resulting from errors in DNA replication was quickly supported by experiments that showed that certain base pairs in a chain of nucleotides bind more strongly together than other base pairs. In essence, parts of a piece of DNA—specifically those strands containing large numbers of adenine-cytosine pairings—formed more stable sections than parts made up of guanine-thymine pairs. Those sections of DNA made up of A-C base pairs are better able to accurately duplicate themselves and so are less prone to replication errors than segments of DNA with an excess of G-T bases.

Indeed, cancer researchers have found that both radiation and carcinogens more easily damaged DNA composed of a majority of G-T base pairings. Sickle cell disease, a severe and at times lethal form of anemia, results from a single base pair change: specifically the substitution of a thymine for a guanine in the gene that should produce a normal hemoglobin molecule.

But from the very moment of discovery of the structure of DNA, the real issue was how an array of only four purine and pyrimidine bases, tightly stacked inside two strands of linked deoxyribose sugars, tucked away within a nucleus, securely locked behind the nuclear membrane, in the center of a cell, could direct the whole of evolution and functioning of all life. In short, how did a sequence of adenines and thymines, guanines and cytosines take life out of chemistry and into the world. Scientists have agreed for decades on the basic physical substance of life. Whatever their religious, professional, or personal beliefs, biologists agree that the fundamental building blocks of all living things, whether nuclear membranes, cell walls, cilia that propel algae, or the muscles that drive a racehorse are all proteins. In essence, it is the ability to produce proteins that gave life its physical basis, its very touch and feel. The question, of course, was how did the sequences of four nucleotides transform themselves into the various peptides and proteins that differentiate the hummingbird from the flower.

11

It's not what you don't know that hurts you.
It's what you think you know that ain't so.

SATCHEL PAIGE

Everything that life is and that life does is made up of and done by proteins. Nothing living has ever been discovered that is void of proteins. Skin and bones are proteins. Muscles, cell walls, nails, hooves, tendons, ligaments, hemoglobin, antibodies, strands of seaweed, insulin, growth hormones, enzymes, the retina of the eye, pollen grains, and spider webs are all proteins. There is no movement without proteins; no leaf grows, no flower turns toward the sun, no bee can fly. Proteins are both the glue and substance of life. Early in the study of DNA, one experiment proved that genes were the blueprints of protein synthesis, and that in fact the units of heredity coded for proteins.

Scientists transplanted the nucleus from a cell of one species into the cytoplasm of a cell from another. The proteins produced by the cell were specific for the species of the transplanted nucleus. Change the nuclei and you change the proteins. The nuclei transfer experiments proved that while the code lay in the nucleus, the protein-making machinery was out in the cytoplasm. It did not take the researchers long to realize that for cells to function somehow the code had to be transferred out of the nucleus into the cell's cytoplasm. Whatever the code turned out to be, it had to be able to get out of the nucleus and physically travel into the cytoplasm to tell the cell exactly what proteins to make.

The scientists did have one important fact to guide them. No matter how complicated or intricate a protein, it is composed of a string of amino acids, the uniqueness of each protein determined by the types of amino acids making up its structure. Moreover there are only twenty-two amino acids available for construction, only twenty-two amino acids survived the original chemical soup. Nature could clearly only work with what it had and so would the scientists.

Once it became clear that the genetic code lay in the sequence of the four different bases lying inside a strand of DNA and that the code, in order to direct protein synthesis, had to direct the arrangement of the different twenty-two amino acids making up each specific protein, the mathematicians were able to get into the act. The simplest mathematical association would have been one base—an adenine, a cytosine, a thymine, or a guanine—matching up with one amino acid. But with twenty-two different amino acids to control, each base would have to code for at least five different amino acids, making it impossible for the blueprint to tell the machinery in the cytoplasm which of the five amino acids controlled by that one base to insert at any specific spot during the synthesis of the protein. A two-base system was again a potential for disaster, garbling the blueprint beyond any hope of cytoplasmic recognition. The only reasonable code was one where each of the twenty-two amino acids had its own base sequence so that the cytoplasm's protein-producing machinery would know precisely which amino acid was coded for at that specific spot in the protein. Hematologists already knew that the replacement of a single amino acid, valine for glycine, in the 300-amino-acid-long alpha chain of the hemoglobin molecule caused life-threatening sickle cell anemia. Multicellular life had become so intricate and exact that nature simply could not become casual about how its proteins were produced. A cellular blueprint without a one-to-one correlation between the genetic code and each of the body's twenty-two amino acids would be like having plans to build a house that read: "At this point, use either a one-inch, one-half–inch, or three-inch bolt."

Mathematically, the minimal grouping of four different bases to code for each one of twenty-two available amino acids is three. Knowing that nature is never more extravagant than necessary, the scientists looked for a code based on a sequence of three bases, in essence a trinary code where each set of three bases along a strand of DNA code for the placement of a specific amino acid along a protein chain. Scientists were willing to bet that nature, for all its apparent diversity, had taken the simplest of all mathematical paths; and they were correct. Early in evolution nature, in assembling its basic structures, used a three-based sequence of nucleotides as the genetic code, linking each three-base sequence with a specific amino acid.

A gene, Mendel's original unit of heredity, is no more and no less than the array of three-base pairs in a strand of DNA.

12

*You're wrestling with a champ. You're trying to
find out how God made the world, just like
Jacob wrestling with an angel.*

I.I. RABI (PHYSICIST)

At the same time that the soon-to-be-called AIDS epidemic was
beginning in Europe and North America the molecular biologists, working on their own and using the new techniques of
ultracentrifugation, protein gel electrophoresis, and xenon radiog-
raphy, were focusing down on how individual cells produce peptides and proteins. The histologists of the nineteenth century
had discovered all kinds of granules floating in the cytoplasm of
cells, from those of bacteria to human tissues, noticing that cytoplasm of more complicated single-celled organisms and the
cells of organs that secrete large amounts of materials contained
more of these granules than cells from less active tissues. Later
biologists found that the granules were protein factories where
polypeptides and proteins are assembled in a stepwise manner,
one amino acid at a time. These cytoplasmic granules were given
the name ribosomes.

Very close to the time the molecular geneticists were realizing that there had to be a method for getting the code out of the nucleus and into the ribosomes, the physicians at San Francisco General Hospital and California Irwin Memorial Blood Bank began to examine past records of the increasing number of patients admitted to Bay area hospitals suffering from weight loss, diarrhea, enlarged lymph nodes, lung infections, and a strange, rare skin cancer called Kaposi's sarcoma. A preliminary evaluation indicated that a number of these patients had been given blood transfusions or blood products in the preceding four years. When the physicians made a more detailed search of blood bank records they found that the donor for a number of the patients was a socially prominent international trade consultant who had recently died of encephalitis.

While the physicians in San Francisco pursued their own mystery, the molecular geneticists found the "messenger" that physically carried the blueprint for protein production out of the nucleus into the cytoplasm. The messenger was discovered to be a small, single strand of the nucleic acid RNA in which a ribose sugar had replaced the deoxyribose of DNA. RNA is not a double helix but a single strand of linked ribose nucleotides; the four bases, though, were the same as in DNA with the exception that a new purine, uracil, had replaced the DNA's cytosine.

The scientists showed that "messenger RNA" was put together in the nucleus from the cell's DNA; each nucleotide base of the messenger was an exact replica of the sequence of the DNA bases, so that the specific coding sequence of a strand of DNA was maintained within the messenger.

During the years that scientists were discovering messenger RNA, two patients in Florida being treated for hemophilia were admitted to the hospital with pneumonia caused by a strange intracellular bacterium called *Pneumocystis carinii*. The Florida physicians were unable to find a reason for a type of pneumonia that was known only to occur in patients on chemotherapy or with a depressed immune system. The physicians wondered if the intravenous blood products given to treat the patient's hemophilia had not become contaminated with the *Pneumocystis* microbe. They reported their concerns to the Centers for Disease Control in Atlanta. Within six months of the first Florida reports of hemophiliacs acquiring pneumocystis lung infections, dozens of other hematologists were finding the same strange infection in their patients. The infectious disease experts at the Centers for Disease Control wondered, too, if the plasma concentrates given to hemophiliacs to replace their own missing clotting factors might not be involved. They became less concerned when they discovered that the last purification procedure used in the production of the pooled plasma was the passage of the plasma through a fine porcelain filter that strained out anything larger than a cell, removing all molds and fungi and bacteria from the final product, clearly eliminating any microorganism from the final concentrate, including any single-celled *Pneumocystis carinii* protozoa. But there were others, more clinicians than researchers, who decided to ignore the accepted view of microbial contamination and rely instead on what they saw and the patients they examined.

An immunologist in New York City giving a lecture on strange infections at a national infectious disease conference presented the case history of a child born to an intravenous drug user. After a protracted illness characterized by weight loss, recurrent ear infections, and fungal infections of the mouth and posterior pharynx, the infant had died of meningitis a few months before his second birthday. When the child was seventeen months of age a bone marrow biopsy had been performed and the microorganism *Mycobacterium avium-intracellulare* had been discovered growing deep in the child's marrow. The child had not been born with any known defect of his immune system; the child had not been treated with any medication known to lower resistance to infection; nor, as was pointed out at the conference, had the child received any blood transfusions or blood products. But what the immunologist found most troubling was that, up until that time, the *M. avium-intracellulare* bacteria had only been found in diseased birds; never, as far as he determined, had the infection been reported in a human. There was clearly something bad going on, but all anyone had was bits and pieces. There was no way, yet, to put it all together.

There is a great concern today about statistics, which is the science of organized observation. It is true that "garbage in" will mean "garbage out" and that large enterprises like the tobacco industry can hire their own so-called experts to obfuscate and confuse the public about observations that are not only reliable but predictive. More to the point, accurate statistics in themselves don't lie. Science, at its best, is nonauthoritarian; it is based on data and experiments that should and, if accurate, will stand on their own, with the author or authors clearly hidden from view. Statistics give science a brutal and at times contentious intellectual distance, and in the middle of the nineteenth century statistics came to medicine. Edmund Snow, an epidemiologist, using residential street maps, charted the spread of the 1854 London cholera epidemic. Snow documented that the disease spread in concentric circles from a single central point, that central point being the Broad Street water pump. The pump supplied the majority of the water for the southwest district of London. Snow presented his maps to public officials along with what he considered the only possible conclusion, that cholera resulted from drinking water drawn from the Broad Street pump.

The English politicians and the London businessmen, supported by a less than enlightened medical establishment, were outraged at Snow's report, not to mention his maps. The water delivered by the Broad Street pump came from the Thames, and the very idea of good English drinking water causing disease was not only unthinkable and un-British but a potential economic disaster. The Thames was used by hundreds of restaurants and thousands of businesses. A general panic was considered to be of no use to anyone, especially if based on no more than a map drawn by some obscure statistician. The stalwarts of the British establishment, assisted by the professors of medicine, happily pointed out the inconsistencies of Snow's data. There were clearly a great number of residences well within Snow's concentric circles that had been spared the disease, as well as the occasional isolated house miles away from the pump where cholera had occurred. These anomalies were used to mock the tidiness of Snow's conclusions. Today we know that those disease-free homes near the pump were the homes of people who had either boiled their water or simply drank beer, while those affected homes well beyond Snow's circles were the homes of families whose members had contracted the disease in residences or businesses closer to the pump or had carried contaminated water back to their own houses. But cholera is a terribly dramatic disease. There is almost no time between infection and symptoms; diarrhea and cramping begin almost immediately. Husbands left for work in the morning and arrived back home at night to find their children incoherent with 105-degree fevers and their wives pleading for help in pools of their own bloody diarrhea. Ten thousand Londoners eventually contracted the disease, and as the epidemic continued and the number of deaths grew, the people of London demanded first that something be done and then, finally, that anything be done.

Pressured to act, the city government eventually had no choice but to listen to Snow and act on the data they had worked so hard to discredit. Six weeks into the epidemic, amidst the angry shouts of the pubic, the city fathers, finally worried more about their jobs than the potential financial damage to both British prestige and commerce, closed down the Broad Street pump and stopped the epidemic.

In quite a real and personal way the people living in London in 1854 were lucky. Cholera was and still is an immediate and devastating disease. Politicians charged with the duty to protect public health are forced to act. There are still epidemics of cholera, but today there is no hesitation; governments quickly close down restaurants, stop the production of potentially contaminated products, and truck in bottled water, whatever the costs.

By the beginning of the 1980s, there had been enough reports of strange infections in supposedly healthy patients for a number of European and American physicians to go through medical records using Snow's statistical techniques and convince themselves that whatever was happening was infectious and was spread from person to person by contaminated blood products, sexual activity, and intravenous drug use. And worse, there appeared to be a long incubation period between infection and symptoms. But few listened. In truth, the long incubation gave public health administrators, blood bank officials, senators, congressmen, a large number of physicians, religious leaders, and even gay activists the time to ignore the disease and worse, to follow their own agendas rather than to look to the public safety.

Even today, in virtually every town and city in America, politicians faced with desperate people dying horrible nightmarish deaths refuse to do what the politicians of London in the 1850s were finally forced to do: look, observe, and act.

But nowhere has this blindness and self-serving been more clearly shown than in the spread of AIDS in children. In February of 1983, at the beginning of the epidemic, a child was admitted to San Francisco's General Hospital because of severe diarrhea and weight loss. Microbial testing showed the child to be infected with cryptosporidiosis, an infection thought to be a disease of domesticated sheep. The physician had no idea what antibiotic might prove to be effective. On a hunch, one of the doctors tracked down the world's expert on cryptosporidiosis, a professor of veterinary medicine at the University of Iowa. The professor was familiar with the *Cryptosporidium* parasite but was surprised when he was asked about treatment. "Treatment?" he answered, "There is no treatment. We shoot the animals."

A decade into the epidemic, infants and children have become one of the largest high-risk groups. Still, physicians in the 1980s struggled to apply common sense and statistics to the whole issue of AIDS while their associates in the more basic science of molecular biology continued their own research into cellular function in the hopes of unraveling what it was that made AIDS so deadly.

The molecular biologists, continuing to work backward from the ribosomes to messenger RNA to DNA, became aware that a step was missing. How did each of the twenty amino acids know where to go? This time the biochemists came to the rescue, specifically, the amino acid specialists. In analyzing the molecular composition of cytoplasm they had found that as soon as one of the twenty-two amino acids enters a cell, it is quickly connected to a free-floating three-base nucleic acid. Each amino acid—lysine, tyrosine, or phenylalanine—has its own specific three-base nucleotide carrier. Indeed, every amino acid entering a cell is not only linked up and transported around the cell by its own "carrier nucleotide," but the sequence of bases in each carrier precisely matches the three-base sequence of the cell's DNA as well as its strand of messenger RNA, guaranteeing the placement of that specific amino acid in its correct location during the production of peptides and proteins.

The discovery of these carrier nucleotides filled in the final gap in what was clearly an age-old transfer of information, begun over 3.5 million years ago when replicating polymers first entered the world of complexity and change.

It seems almost fanciful to think that underneath, everything works the same. Yet there has always been that subliminal, poetic sense in all of us that despite outward diversity, there exists a sameness and connectedness that allows cows to eat the same corn we eat, insects to be drawn to the same flowers that we enjoy, and the songbird's song to echo within each of us. This commonality of life, the sense that for better or for worse we are all connected, was brought into the general consciousness by one man whose genius and creativity allowed him to bridge that world of science and of art.

13

The enemy of my enemy is my friend.

MUSLIM PROVERB

It was Louis Pasteur who was to prove that there is a basic fundamental identity of all living things. Pasteur started his scientific career by solving what was at the time one of chemistry's most enduring enigmas. It had been discovered in 1844 that certain carbon compounds, specifically the crystals of sodium-ammonium paratartrate, with identical chemical compositions, equal molecular weights, and precisely the same physical properties, including duplicate melting and freezing points, would when dissolved in solution cause a polarized light to rotate in exactly opposite directions. The discontinuous shifting of polarized light by two supposedly identical carbon compounds troubled the world's chemists. The fact that molecules that were apparently exactly the same could produce such diametrically opposite physical effects was of great concern because it meant that the scientists were missing something fundamental about these compounds and perhaps something fundamental about nature itself. And as it turned out, they were correct in their concerns.

Pasteur attacked the problem of the so called "Mitscherlich

planes" with a commitment and attention to detail that was to become his trademark for the remainder of his scientific career. He began by first synthesizing the crystals of paratartrates himself and then dissolving the crystals in water, proving to himself that the liquid was absolutely neutral in the presence of polarized light. He then boiled off the liquid and, when the crystals reformed, withdrew individual crystals from the mother fluid. He found under a microscope that two types of crystals had formed, each the exact mirror image of the other. Pasteur could actually separate the crystals into the two different types, which he called "right- and left-handed." When he redissolved only right-handed crystals, the solution rotated polarized light to the right; when he made a solution of only left-handed crystals and passed the same polarized light through the left-handed solution, the light was rotated 180 degrees opposite the rotation of the right-handed solution.

Pasteur considered the discovery to be so important that thirty years after the event, he felt compelled to explain it to students in a lecture he gave to the Société Chimique de Paris.

> I was a student at the Ecole Normale Supérieure, from 1843 to 1846. Chance made me read in the school library a note of the learned crystallographer, Mitscherlich, related to two salts: the tartrate and the paratartrate of sodium and ammonium. I meditated for a long time upon this note; it disturbed my schoolboy thoughts. I could not understand that two substances could be as similar as claimed by Mitscherlich, without being completely identical. To know how to wonder and question is the first step of the mind toward discovery.
>
> Hardly graduated from the Ecole Normale, I planned to prepare a long series of crystals, with the purpose of studying their shapes. I selected tartaric acid and its salts, as well as paratartaric acid, for the following reasons. The crystals of all these substances are as beautiful as they are easy to prepare. On the other hand, I could constantly control the accuracy of my determinations by referring to the memoir of an able and very precise physicist,

M. de la Provostaye, who had published an extensive crystallo-graphic study of tartaric and paratartaric acid and of their salts.

I soon recognized that . . . tartaric acid and all its combinations exhibit asymmetric forms. Individually, each of these forms of tartaric acid gave a mirror image which was not superposable upon the substance itself. On the contrary, I could not find anything of the sort in paratartaric acid or its salts.

Suddenly, I was seized by a great emotion. I had always kept in mind the profound surprise caused in me by Mitscherlich's note on the tartrate and paratartrate of sodium and ammonium. Despite the extreme thoroughness of their study, I thought, Mitscherlich, as well as M. de la Provostaye, will have failed to notice that the tartrate is asymmetric, as it must be; nor will they have seen that the paratartrate is not asymmetric, which is also very likely. Immediately, and with a feverish ardor, I prepared the double tartrate of sodium and ammonium, as well as the corresponding paratartrate, and proceeded to compare their crystalline forms, with the preconceived notion that I would find asymmetry in the tartrate and not in the paratartrate. Thus, I thought, everything will become clear, the mystery of Mitscherlich's note will be solved, the asymmetry in the form of the tartrate crystal will correspond to its optical asymmetry, and the absence of asymmetry in the form of the paratartrate will correspond to the inability of this salt to deviate the plane of polarized light. . . . And indeed, I saw that the crystals of the tartrates of sodium and ammonium exhibited the small facets revealing asymmetry; but when I turned to examine the shape of the crystals of paratartrate, for an instant my heart stopped beating: all the crystals exhibited the facets of asymmetry!

The fortunate idea came to me to orient my crystals with reference to a plane perpendicular to the observer, and then I noticed that the confused mass of crystals of paratartrate could be divided into two groups according to the orientation of their facets of asymmetry. In one group, the facet of asymmetry nearer my body was inclined to my right with reference to the plane of orientation which I just mentioned, whereas the facet of asymmetry was inclined to my left in the other. The paratartrate appeared as a mixture of two kinds of crystals, some asymmetric to the right, some asymmetric to the left.

A new and obvious idea soon occurred to me. These crystals

asymmetric to the right, which I could separate manually from the others, exhibited an absolute identity of shape with those of the classical right tartrate. Pursuing my preconceived idea, in the logic of its deductions, I separated these right crystals from the crystallized paratartrate; I made the lead salt and isolated the acid; this acid appeared absolutely identical with the tartaric acid of grape, identical also in its action on polarized light. My happiness was even greater the day when, separating now from the paratartrate the crystals with asymmetry at their left, and making their acid, I obtained a tartaric acid absolutely similar to the tartaric acid of grape, but with an opposite asymmetry, and also with an opposite action on light. Its shape was identical to that of the mirror image of the right tartaric acid and, other things being equal, it rotated light to the left as much in absolute amount as the other acid did it to the right.

"It was indeed evident," Pasteur wrote in his memoirs, "that the strongest light had been thrown on the cause of the phenomena of rotary polarization, when a new class of isomeric substances was discovered; the unexpected and until then unexplained constitution of the paratartric acid was revealed."

Pasteur's discovery that organic molecules, while identical in virtually every measurable way, could still be produced in two opposite three-dimensional configurations took the science of chemistry into the third dimension and Pasteur into the sciences of biology and medicine. Pasteur wondered if he might not have discovered a basic property true of all organic molecules, namely, that organic substances can be produced in two, dimensionally opposite forms. He began to study other organic compounds and indeed discovered that there was this fundamental distinction between organic and inorganic chemistry. All organic molecules synthesized in the laboratory did have this right- and left-handedness, a property that was not a part of compounds not containing carbon. But Pasteur also made another discovery that was equally intriguing, specifically that despite synthetic organic compounds being produced in different three-dimensional forms, the organic molecules produced by living things were only produced in one form. Pasteur checked and rechecked the sugars, alcohols, peptides, and proteins produced by living organisms and found that they were all three-dimensionally left-handed.

Very early in evolution, nature was faced with two possible alternatives and chose one and stayed with that choice, from single-celled algae through to the sugars in human cells. Here is clearly a basic, mysterious sameness to all living things, but it is also an indication of a strange internal fragility, which became tragically evident when in the 1960s a German pharmaceutical company produced a new sedative that was said to have no major complications.

Today it appears that the synthetically produced thalidomide, a sedative taken by pregnant women that caused their children to be born with absent or malformed arms and legs, is a 50–50 mixture of left- and right-handed optical isomers. It is now proposed that the right-handed molecule is close enough in structure to its biologically active but embryonically benign left-handed sister that both substances are readily absorbed by a fetus; but that once inside the developing cells, the right-handed molecule, like a wrongly threaded screw or bolt, so disrupts the inner workings of the fetal cells that those cells programed to become the future limbs of the fetus are poisoned and never develop properly.

Recently organic chemists have found that the synthetic production of psychoactive drugs, including the antidepressant fluoxetine hydrochloride, results in the production of both right- and left-handed molecules. Researchers now worry that the undesirable side effects of these drugs, the paranoia and suicidal tendencies, result from the exposure of brain cells to the right-handed disruptive isomer. One investigator recently wrote, ". . . life inside a cell is under the control of exquisitely precise enzymes and receptors that fit their targets like a hand in a glove. For the most part, the right-handed drug does not fit into a left-handed receptor or enzyme [systems]."

Pasteur's discovery of the left-handedness of life's molecules had a profound effect on the world's understanding of evolution. It proved what was slowly becoming evident: whatever life's outward complexity, down in its basic machinery, where peptides, sugars, nucleotides, and enzymes have to combine and interact, we are indeed all the same, using the identical left-handed fasteners, gears, screws, nuts, and bolts.

A perfect example of how outer shapes can disguise life's internal identities occurred first in the seas of the Cambrian era. It is obvious from the fossil records that diversity took an enormous leap forward a little over half a billion years ago. In the preceding billion years while photosynthesis was filling the atmosphere with oxygen there had been a slow, progressive evolution of multicellular jellyfish and soft-bodied tubular wormlike creatures from the original single-celled organisms. Then within less than 100 million years, a blink in geologic time, body forms changed and the waters of the Cambrian age erupted in strange and varied animals. The world's first monsters appeared: *Anomalocaris*, with great bulging eyes and grasping, tearing claws, its body taking on the aspects of both stingray and lobster. Teeth appeared and hard, calcium-encrusted plates formed armorlike outer shells.

Within a few million years of the entry of *Anomalocaris* into the world's oceans, all the different body designs seen on earth today came into existence. *Naraoia* acquired the ability to use sensory antennae. *Fuxianhuia* used its antennae to house developing eye parts, giving this genus an edge in the hunting of other genera. *Jianfengia* developed sharp appendages, while the jointed legs of the hard-shelled trilobites quickly turned into gills. The whole family of Hallucigenia, with its array of needle-sharp spinets, suddenly emerged full blown next to *Anomalocaris*, beside its close cousin, *Microdicyton*, with its huge crushing jaws, while the carnivorous worm, *Ottoia*, sped along the ocean floor snapping up prey through its new whiplike mouth.

Life during the Cambrian era appeared to become an ever-escalating arms race, new defenses giving way to new means of attack, better defenses being overwhelmed by the development of an ever more effective and deadly offensive arsenal. The appearance of spines probably caused predators to make their own evolutionary leaps to larger mouths. But the single major genetic transition that seemed to fuel this amazing diversity was the evolution from soft bodies to hard shells, spines to gills, and scales to strong, rigid exoskeletons.

Yet all this development may have been no more than the effects of adding a new element, calcium carbonate, to the seawater. Increasing levels of carbon dioxide occurring in the atmosphere and later in seawater during the early Cambrian period caused calcium in the oceans to precipitate as particles of calcium carbonate. Calcium carbonate can be incorporated into the outer walls of a membrane to form a hard, crusty barrier. A protein in a soft cell wall that could bind particles of calcium carbonate, a small change in the genetic code that slightly altered an already available protein to give it a new binding capacity or three-dimensional shape, allowing the newly revised protein to bind the new molecules of calcium carbonate, would begin a whole new phase shift—a transformation from a soft exterior to a more protective outer covering of hard scales and shells that would give such a survival advantage to this "new" creature that one gene for carbonate binding would be carried forward into the code of the descendants of these more protected animals. The advantage in evolutionary terms of soft-bodied animals suddenly developing a hard exosurface is obvious; the additional advantage offered by internalizing that hard outer surface to create an internal skeleton that was no longer at the mercy of external concentrations of calcium carbonate virtually guaranteed the emergence of creatures with a backbone to evolve alongside their already-armored cousins.

But everything still remained left-handed. The sugars found

in the sap of fossilized trees and in *Anomalocaris* are stereoscopically identical with sugars that Pasteur found in modern plants and animals.

At the time that Pasteur was studying the three-dimensional structures of sugars, the spoilage of food and wine was considered both by the scientific community and the Church to be due to substances called "ferments" that mysteriously entered all food and food products, leading to their inevitable decay and putrefaction. Pasteur became convinced through his studies of organic substances that fermentation was not caused by ferments but occurred quite naturally because bacteria contaminated the food products and used the available sugars for their own energy, and in the process of cellular metabolism changed those sugars into less energy-rich vinegars.

Pasteur presented his theory attributing the process of fermentation to microbial contamination to the French Academy of Sciences. He had the same problem that Bassi had faced earlier in the century. The idea of living substances causing chemical change was not only in direct opposition to the accepted and "chemically correct" theory of ferments, but it also violated the religious doctrine of the spontaneous generation of life, the view that living creatures, bacteria, spores, and single-celled organisms, through God's intervention can and do arise spontaneously from inactive mineral matter. Religious scholars and those in the scientific and quasiscientific community attacked Pasteur and his theory of microbial contamination. The religious enmity generated by Pasteur's attack on spontaneous generation was to follow him for the rest of his life. But science and its methods of quantification had come so far by the 1860s and Pasteur's techniques were so meticulous and his interpretations so focused that his results could not be ignored. Besides, the respect for science had reached a point where industry had become interested in its conclusions.

The French winegrowers, concerned about increasing spoilage and more worried about profits than Church doctrine, asked

Pasteur to apply his new theory of bacterial contamination to their products. Pasteur quickly proved that wine could be prevented from spoiling without loss of taste by gently heating it to between 55 and 60 degrees centigrade, a temperature that he showed destroyed bacteria without damaging the wine's concentrations of sugars, tannins, and complicated alcohols. The heating process, which soon became universal, was eventually called "pasteurization" in honor of Pasteur. Within the year Pasteur was using the same technique to save the German beer industry.

But still Pasteur was challenged on the issue of spontaneous generation until, with one grand experiment, he put to rest once and for all the whole concept of new life evolving where and when it chose. Having devised a hollow, dumbbell-shaped flask, Pasteur placed a piece of meat in one end of the flask, heating that end to pasteurize the meat, at the same time sealing the thin, hollow portion connecting the two ends. He next placed a culture of bacteria in the opposite end of the flask. Pasteur showed that no matter what was done to the meat, no matter how long it was placed in sunlight or buried in the ground, spoilage and the generation of new colonies of bacteria and mold occurred only if the trap between the two portions of the flask was broken and the bacteria were allowed to reach the meat.

This linking of the apparent generation of life to a process that had no need of a divine creator was a construct that put Pasteur at odds not only with the Church but with the accepted view of evolution. Yet it was a position from which Pasteur could not retreat, a thesis that he defended in the simplest of terms: "Neither religion nor philosophy nor atheism nor materialism nor spiritualism has any place here . . . it is a question of fact. I have approached [the issue of spontaneous creation] without preconceived idea."

Pasteur, ignoring his critics, acknowledged his successes as well as what had sustained him by a motto that became famous: Trust in science. He might well have restated Paracelsus's admonition, ". . . to go back to the bedside, to look, and be suspicious of eloquence," to the more modern "go back to the laboratory, look, and be suspicious of eloquence."

Pasteur had been dragged into the world of biology and would have gladly gone back to his beloved chemistry, but fame got in the way. In 1871 he was asked to use his skills to save Europe's poultry industry. Europe's chicken and turkey farms were routinely decimated by chicken cholera, an infectious disease easily spread from bird to bird and flock to flock. Pasteur was asked to do for these farms what he had already done for the wine and beer industries. He agreed and after two years of benchwork, Pasteur was able to isolate the bacterium that caused the disease. He had begun his studies by collecting the diarrheal feces from diseased birds, culturing the feces, and then painstakingly subculturing the bacterial growth until he was able to isolate in pure culture the specific offending microorganism, the chicken cholera bacillus.

It is unclear exactly what Pasteur had planned to do with the vials of pure cultures other than to have a fresh supply of bacteria available for additional studies. Eventually the bacteria growing in the flasks became so thick that they outgrew the medium's nutrients and began to die. Pasteur had to continually transfer a few colonies to newer flasks in order to keep a ready supply of healthy, dividing bacteria. Pasteur was using his cultures to infect a new batch of birds when by mistake he apparently took one of the older, overgrown flasks. The inoculated birds never developed cholera. Pasteur was too great a scientist to ignore the obvious and quickly checked his records and found that he had injected the birds with organisms from an older flask. He examined the bacteria in the flask and found that the majority of the bacteria were alive and appeared quite normal. Pasteur realized that either the healthy birds he had injected were different from all other healthy birds or that something had happened to the bacteria. A few more injections from these "aged" cultures along with controlled injections of new growths of bacteria proved quite remarkably that bacteria from the older cultures did not cause the disease. Pasteur analyzed and reanalyzed his data and concluded that bacteria in aged cultures had somehow, as he wrote in his notebooks, become "weakened" so that when injected into healthy birds, the bacteria would not or could not cause disease.

Then Pasteur did an extraordinary thing, something quite beyond what anyone else had ever done and in all probability beyond what any scientist of the time would even have considered. The mathematician Mark Kac tried once to explain the essence of true intellectual brilliance. "There are two kinds of geniuses," Kac wrote, "the *ordinary* and the *magicians*. An ordinary genius is a fellow that you and I would be just as good as, if we were only many times better. There is no mystery as to how [their] minds work. Once we understand what they have done, we feel certain that we, too, could have done it. It is different with the magicians. They are, to use the mathematical jargon, in the orthogonal complement of where we are and the working of their minds is, for all intents and purposes, incomprehensible. Even after we understand what they have done, the process by which they have done it is completely dark."

Pasteur was a magician. What he did in the silence of his laboratory still baffles everyone who reads his notes. Pasteur took cultures that had not been aged and injected the lethal bacillus into the birds he had *previously* injected with the aged, apparently noninfectious cultures. It was an experiment that changed the world. The doubly injected birds did not go on to develop cholera. The only possible explanation was that injections of the weakened bacteria had somehow protected the birds when they were exposed to the still-virulent strains.

Pasteur, working twenty hours a day, stayed at his workbench until he had convinced himself that the explanation for this protection did not lie in the culture media, the nutrients, or even the bacteria themselves but in some as-yet-unexplained connection between the birds and their previous exposures to the weakened bacillus. Pasteur concluded that the injection of the weakened cholera bacillus was somehow similar to what occurred in humans when vaccinated with Jenner's cowpox. Pasteur presented his discovery of the protection of healthy birds from chicken cholera when first injected with his weakened bacteria to a convention of the European chicken industry and though he could offer no specific explanation for the protection, the breeders needed no prompting. Old cultures of cholera bacillus were used to vaccinate the chicken population of Europe. Within a year, the continent was free of chicken cholera.

Pasteur, more than any scientist of the nineteenth century, understood that science gives universal truths and that, similar to his paratartrates, what he had discovered in his cholera vaccines was something fundamental, unalterable by national boundaries or individual concerns. Koch had cataloged the world of microbiology, but that was only half the task. Pasteur set out to accomplish the second half.

Indeed, Pasteur realized that if he had discovered a universal truth that protection from an infectious disease was offered by preexposure to a changed or weakened bacterium, then he should be able to protect cows from anthrax by injecting aged anthrax cultures into susceptible herds. But it didn't work and worse, virtually all those animals inoculated with overgrown and aged cultures went on to develop anthrax.

But then Pasteur did a second magical thing, an action so beyond reason and perhaps even thought that then or now no one could have anticipated or explained his actions. He killed the anthrax in his cultures with phenol. Why Pasteur considered that dead bacteria, indeed that anything dead, would work in a biological setting was all part of the magic. He then took the cultures to which he had added phenol and injected the dead bacteria into his control group of healthy animals. When these newly "vaccinated" animals were exposed to the spores of the anthrax bacillus, none became infected. In protecting the cows of Europe Pasteur had conjured up the first killed bacterial vaccine. All later human vaccines—diphtheria, pertussis, rubella, mumps, chicken pox, and influenza—are, even today, based on the methods and techniques that Pasteur devised to produce his anthrax vaccine.

Pasteur had indeed discovered something quite fundamental—even more fundamental than he could have anticipated. His vaccines proved once and for all that all living things are indeed similar and that at some basic physiological level they all do know each other and, perhaps more astonishing, that the fight for survival does not depend on whether an attacking microorganism is alive or dead.

Over the next twenty years, Pasteur's germ theory of disease and Koch's microbial techniques became the dominant force in medicine. Bacteria were sought as the cause of all kinds of disease. This emphasis on infection in medicine proved so powerful that for a time the idea that all disease was caused by invading bacteria threatened to overrun all aspects of medical care. Yet there were a number of diseases that were clearly infectious for which no offending bacterium or microorganism could be found either in water, in the air, or in the patients themselves.

In laboratories throughout the world physicians struggled to identify the bacteria in patients with measles, mumps, chicken pox, and rabies, the one clearly infectious disease that was 100 percent fatal. No human bitten by a rabid animal ever survived even though, despite repeated cultures, no bacteria were found.

Some clinical aspects of rabies, though, were clear even though no bacteria were found. The disease was not spread through the air or by simple contact with a rabid animal. One had to be bitten, but once a person had been bitten, the symptoms and course of the illness were always the same. Within a week or two the patient would begin to experience a change in personality. Soon there would be fever, tremors, hallucinations followed by seizures, and then paralysis, and ultimately death.

The lethality of rabies, the terror and hopelessness of those bitten, and the prolonged and brutal dying was feared throughout the world. The cry of "rabid dog" was enough to clear the streets of any city or town and send the people of whole villages running back into their homes.

Pasteur's vaccines began a great debate in biology. The idea of physically altering disease-causing bacteria or killing them to be used as vaccines was not only new but a bewildering concept. How could you propose a theory and then implement it without having the slightest idea how it worked? Still, in the real world, results count; it was only a matter of time before Pasteur was asked to apply his theories to treating human disease.

In 1878 Pasteur, prompted by his medical colleagues, was asked to try to find a vaccine for rabies. Pasteur reluctantly agreed and took up the challenge, doing what he always did, going back to the laboratory and starting at the beginning. He began his study of rabies with what he already knew about bacteria and once again leaving his beloved chemistry behind, he reported in 1881 that rabies was not caused by a bacillus but by a new kind of infectious substance that he found to exist in the saliva of rabid animals. Since rabies was caused only by a bite, Pasteur had directed his attention to the rabid animal's saliva. Carefully using Koch's techniques, he had cultured saliva but found no microorganisms. Yet when he injected that same saliva into a healthy animal, the animal inevitably developed rabies.

In order to prove that he was not missing a bacterium that simply would not grow in his different broths, Pasteur added a new step to the study of microbiology and ultimately added to the basic understanding of evolution itself. Pasteur strained the supposedly infectious saliva through a fine porcelain filter. He had measured the pores of the filters and was confident that the openings were physically too small to allow the passage of any known bacterium, much less a portion of any living tissue including individual cells. No bacteria could possibly pass through the fine pores of his filters; and yet the material he collected

below the filter from rabies-producing saliva were still as infectious as unstrained saliva. With characteristic simplicity, Pasteur named the infectious material that had so obviously passed
through the pores a "filterable agent," and continued with his
experiments.

Pasteur focused his attention on the filtered saliva or, more
accurately, on what the filtered but infectious material did,
namely, cause rabies.

Since rabid animals first became disoriented and then had
seizures, Pasteur began to examine the brains of diseased animals using the same techniques he had used on the samples of
saliva. He filtered parts of the supposedly infected brains and,
using the materials below the filters, found that his infectious
"filterable agent" did indeed exist in the brain tissues of rabid
animals and did indeed continue to pass through his porcelain
filters. But how had the rabid material infected the brain? Pasteur understood that clinically there was the well-established
time gap between being bitten by a rabid animal and the beginning of the disease. Pasteur questioned his medical colleagues
about the progression of symptoms and found that the length of
time between a bite and the beginning of the dementia and
seizures seemed to depend on the closeness of the bite to the patient's brain. Bites around the head and neck led to death within
hours; bites on the legs and arms might lead to a number of perfectly healthy days before the beginning of symptoms. Pasteur
began a more detailed and meticulous postmortem dissection of
rabid animals and, examining all the tissues in the same way he
had examined diseased brains, found the filterable agent traveled
up the peripheral nerves of the infected animals but existed only
in nerves coming from the immediate area of the bite. Pasteur
went on to do timed dissections, where after injections of rabid
saliva the animals were sacrificed at specific intervals of lapsed
time and found that his filterable agent gradually progressed up
the nerves to the spinal cord and from the spinal cord directly up
into the nerve cells of the brain. If the bite was in an extremity,

the infectious material might take days to reach the brain. The filterable agent quite literally marched slowly up the nerve roots from the site of exposure. Pasteur assumed that the length of time between a bite and the beginning of symptoms had to do with the time it took the filterable agent to reach the cells of the central nervous system. He proved his theory by finding he could produce rabies almost instantaneously in experimental animals by injecting the infected saliva directly into the brain.

Applying what he had learned from his cholera and anthrax vaccines, Pasteur hoped to weaken the infectious material by injecting his filtered substance into different species, waiting a day, and then removing and drying the nervous tissues. He then planned to use the dried tissue as a vaccine, hoping that drying the tissue would alter the agent, making it less lethal but still able to protect the animals from any exposure to the wild strain. He injected the dried neural tissue extracts from infected rabbits into healthy dogs. He then placed these "immunized" dogs along with noninjected animals into cages with rabid animals. All the dogs were bitten, but only the dogs treated with his extracts survived. Whatever the cause of rabies, the drying had weakened the agent and protected his immunized animals.

Pasteur suggested that as a public health measure all the dogs of Europe be vaccinated with his new vaccine. The idea was accepted, but fate would push Pasteur far beyond advocating immunization of animals. Pasteur never considered using his vaccine on humans, but the news of his vaccine soon spread throughout Europe, and in the fall of 1885 a mother brought her child to Pasteur's laboratory begging for his help. Her son, a nine-year-old shepherd boy, had been bitten by a rabid wolf. Pasteur agreed to examine the boy and found fourteen bites on the child's arms and legs. His vaccine had only been given to dogs *before* they had been bitten, while this boy was clearly already infected. The issue, of course, was whether his vaccine would protect someone who had already been exposed to a rabies infection. In short, would his methods be applicable to a human bitten by a rabid animal, but still in the incubation stage of the disease. Pasteur was well aware that he had not performed the experiments necessary to prove or disprove that exposure to his vaccine would be effective following a bite from a rabid animal. And, of course, there was the issue of whether the weakened material might not itself cause the disease in humans as his original weakened anthrax vaccine had caused anthrax in cows. Pasteur considered waiting until the child showed the first symptoms of the disease, but by then, according to his own data, it would in all probability be already too late. If there were to be any hope at all, his vaccine would have to be administered before the infectious material reached the child's brain. Pasteur's beloved science was the only hope.

Pasteur had no idea how his filterable agent caused the dementia and ultimate death of a rabid animal or person, though he was confident that in order for the disease to occur, the infectious agent did indeed have to enter the patient's nerves and work its way up into the neurons of the brain. The real issue was whether there was time for the vaccine to work in a person already exposed.

Unable to ignore the pleas of the mother and faced with the certain death of the child, Pasteur disregarded the advice of the more prudent of his friends and the warnings and veiled threats of his enemies regarding the inappropriateness of a chemist treating human beings with unproven substances. Pasteur started with serial dilutions of his rabbit vaccine, giving daily injections of increasing potency. The world waited, a little boy and his mother waited, and medicine waited.

"I could not sleep the night before the last injection," Pasteur wrote. "The material I was using was so deadly, so undiluted, that it killed an unprotected dog in less than a day."

It is a matter of medical record that the boy survived and even today Pasteur's fame reaches into the hearts and hopes of anyone bitten by a rabid animal.

14

A ship in port is safe,
but that is not what ships are made for.

PROVERB

The word *virus* was used for the first time in 1898. In the fall of that year a Dutch botanist, Martinus Beijerinck, rather reluctantly admitted that a number of plant blights could only result in the passage from plant to plant of an infectious material that was not a bacterium and, more ominously, that simply could not be found or grown outside of the diseased plants. Beijerinck called this infectious material a *virus*, Latin for "poison."

Pasteur and Beijerinck had each been baffled in their own way by what they had discovered, led astray by the basic assumption of evolution that the fundamental unit of life was the cell. It is a prejudice that continues today.

In 1982 an article in the *Morbidity and Mortality Weekly Report* described for the first time what was later to become known as the AIDS epidemic. The article chronicled a number of case histories of patients, excluding hemophiliacs, presenting to their physicians with chronic diarrhea, skin tumors, and a number of strange and unexplained infections.

Two things were made clear by the article. The first was the extraordinarily high mortality of these patients, reflecting as the authors wrote, ". . . the severity of the illness as well as the general debilitation of many of these men"; the second, somewhat less specific but just as accurate, was that when these patients were looked at as a group, all had been ill for weeks to months with fevers and diarrhea, and early in their illness they all developed a general increase in the size of their lymph nodes well before they came to a physician's attention.

The authors observed that while the patients reported in the article had come from over fifteen different states, the District of Columbia, and two foreign countries, well over three-fourths were homosexual men from New York City, San Francisco, and Los Angeles, and that apparently as a group, the homosexual population was at greatest risk. "Although it is possible," the authors wrote, "that the concentration of reported Kaposi's sarcoma, pneumocystis pneumonias, and other opportunistic infections among homosexual men living in New York and California represents a reporting artifact, we consider this possibility unlikely." In truth it was a strange time, when scientists felt obliged to downplay observations and gently disparage their own conclusions. They should have quoted Paracelsus and Frascatorius, Jenner and Semmelweis, ". . . open your eyes, look and believe what you see."

The African and European physicians, having been drawn into the epidemic earlier, were not as interested or obsessed with the apparent homosexual nature of the disease as were their American colleagues. It was not that they challenged the North American data on the numbers of homosexuals presenting with symptoms, but they were simply mystified with the North American preoccupation with the homosexuality instead of the disease. The African and European doctors viewed the high incidence of homosexuals as only a sideshow, real but a statistical quirk, not so much a matter of concern about sexual preference as about numbers of partners. When the European researchers working with their African colleagues began their own investigation they started their evaluations in the remote villages along Lake Victoria where the disease appeared to have begun. They quickly discovered that the disease had initially appeared only in villagers who were sexually active, almost exclusively husbands and wives. Older aunts and uncles, grandparents, and sexually inactive teenagers had been spared. The African physicians and their English colleagues at the London Tropical Disease Institute were convinced early in their investigation that the illness was sexually transmitted. The Europeans viewed the American emphasis on homosexuality as a foolish and unnecessary distraction. It has been said that many of America's politicians, infectious disease experts, and some virologists concerned about political correctness initially refused to pursue the cause of AIDS vigorously because of the early emphasis on the homosexual nature of the disease.

A recent survey of sexual activity of Americans gives a reason for the apparent differences in the type of sexual activity that spread AIDS in Africa as opposed to that in the cities of North America. It appears that heterosexual Americans simply don't have intercourse at the same rate or with as many partners as Africans. A study entitled *Sex in America* (see reference list) reported that one-third of all married couples do not have intercourse during any one year, while another one-third have only occasional sex. The number of extramarital affairs does not keep pace with rates expressed in the tabloids; less than 15 percent of married women and approximately 20 percent of married men admit to having had an extramarital affair. Given that the most adventurous of America's heterosexuals have fewer than ten partners during a lifetime, sexual activity among America's heterosexuals is a rather tame affair. African culture permits more male infidelity and, while not equaling the enormous numbers of sexual encounters that occurred in the homosexual bathhouses of the 1970s and 1980s, the numbers were sufficient and the opportunities frequent enough for a clever sexually transmitted virus to spread through a susceptible population. This was not a new phenomenon. The incidence of syphilis, gonorrhea, and herpes are all related to absolute degrees of sexual activity.

The African physicians had experience with a number of sexually transmitted diseases as well as a series of devastating, though limited, epidemics that had occurred earlier in the decade. But in those epidemics occurring along the Ebola River and in the Great Rift Valley of central Africa, those infected died. Most of the villagers affected died within days, suffering from hemorrhaging and kidney and heart failure. What was stunning about this disease was its infectiousness. The physicians and medical staff caring for these patients became ill and like the villagers also soon died, after suffering the same sudden onset of fevers and massive hemorrhaging.

A similar outbreak of a severe hemorrhagic febrile disease had occurred in Marburg, Germany, and in Yugoslavia in the 1960s. In both cases the disease was traced to direct contact with blood, organs, and cell cultures from a batch of African green monkeys that had been trapped in Uganda. The disease in the Ebola valley and Great Rift Valley was indistinguishable from the illness in Yugoslavia and Germany. In both instances there was the abrupt onset of severe frontal and temporal headaches followed by high fever and generalized muscle pain. Many of the patients complained of difficulty breathing and most developed a severe maculopapular skin rash, ulcers of the mouth, and diarrhea. They then became incoherent and started to bleed into their gut and lungs and died within a day. This new epidemic with its slow course was clearly different, though just as deadly.

Years after the Ebola and Marburg epidemics an electron microscopic evaluation of a liver biopsy specimen preserved from one of the dying patients showed a tiny horseshoe-shaped structures inside the cells of the liver.

Plagues have always been a part of human existence. Thucydides, in his history of the Peloponnesian War, wrote in 430 B.C.:

"Those with naturally strong constitutions were no better than the weak to resist the disease, which carried away all alike, even those treated and dieted with greatest care . . . terrible too was the sight of people dying like sheep through having caught the disease as a result of nursing others. . . ." The plague of Athens had started in Ethiopia and spread to Greece and by the end of a year over a quarter of Athens's population had perished. It has not been lost on today's infectious disease experts that the symptoms as presented by Thucydides and the fact that the disease quickly spread to those caring for the ill exactly resemble the course of today's Ebola virus epidemics and may well have been the first documentation of the spread of a retrovirus out of Africa.

Great physicians have always wondered about the connections between things and throughout the 1980s, as the incidence of AIDS increased, infectious disease experts began to wonder about a connection between the Haitians, homosexuals, hemophiliacs, and the African villagers and these and earlier African epidemics.

For hundreds of years, epidemics of leukemia had regularly ravaged the populations of southern Japan. The Japanese physicians, with their usual thoroughness, had charted the distribution and spread of these various epidemics. After rechecking the historical data, the Japanese researchers became convinced that these cancers were caused by a transmissible infectious agent, most likely a virus.

But what really interested the Japanese was that these epidemics of leukemia were restricted geographically to those regions of Japan settled in the fifteenth century by Portuguese traders who, before reaching Japan, had stopped along the coasts of central Africa. It was a stretch, but there were a few virologists who saw an association between the development of AIDS in Africa, its presentation in Haitians, the Portuguese, and the leukemias in Japan and wondered if all of it might not be somehow related.

In truth there was already a great deal of evidence linking tumors, viruses, leukemias, and strange infections, but it was for the most part only in the veterinarian literature.

In 1908 the British biologist Ellermann, using the techniques of Koch and Pasteur to study cancer in animals, proved—at least to his own satisfaction and that of a few other researchers—that a disease in fowl called "lymphomatosis," similar to the human leukemias, was transmitted by a filterable agent. Ellermann had taken the malignant tissues of diseased birds and, after mincing the tissues and squeezing the cells through Pasteur filters, found that when the cell-free solutions collected below the filters were injected back into healthy birds, the birds' lymphocytes eventually underwent a malignant degeneration, producing precisely the same types of leukemia that had been found in the original diseased birds. It was obvious that whatever passed on the malignancy was smaller than a cell and was infectious, though not in the usual sense of causing a devastating febrile illness but rather in causing cancer.

Ellermann's discovery led other scientists to use his techniques to look for filterable agents in other malignancies. Dr. Payton Rous, working in France, found that some types of apparently spontaneous solid animal tumors could be produced in animals by using filterable extracts made from the cancerous tissues. Breast tumors in certain strains of mice were shown to contain filterable agents that would induce tumors in other mice; and, more importantly, this cancer-causing agent was found to be present in the mammary tissue of adult female mice, transmitted from mothers to offspring during nursing. The transferred agent apparently lay dormant for months in the infant mice, causing tumors only as the suckling mice matured.

Leukemias in cats, as well as a preleukemic condition in which the cats acquired strange and unexpected infections, was shown to be caused by still other filterable agents. There had been a great deal of solid scientific research conducted over a period of 150 years available for study when the villagers and physicians in the Ebola and the Rift valleys began to die and later when the hemophiliacs in Florida began to develop pneumocystis lung infections. Unfortunately, as so often happens, these strange ideas about malignancies and epidemics of leukemia and filterable agents were ignored.

The problem was viruses. Viral diseases have always been a problem for medicine, not only in the scientific sense, but both therapeutically and emotionally. Physicians like to do things; they like to treat patients, to do good, to make their patients better, to be helpful and, more important, be useful. But there is nothing to be done for a viral illness. There are no treatments for viral infections, no drainage procedures, no operations, and no antibiotics. There is nothing to be done except to wait for the patient to recover, nothing to do but wait for the hepatitis to resolve, the encephalitis to disappear, or the myocarditis to heal itself, hardly an appealing scenario to any physician, particularly a modern-day physician working with high-priced, high-tech medical equipment.

Viruses are not bacteria. They aren't even cells. Jenner had never understood what it was in the extracts from cowpox that protected against smallpox, nor did Pasteur quite work out the cause of rabies. The ability to see viruses and prove to everyone's satisfaction that they existed and caused disease had to await the discovery of the electron microscope. But good science can always overcome poor eyesight, and both Jenner and Pasteur, without seeing what was there, understood that they were dealing with real physical objects obeying real physical laws, clearly causing real diseases.

There was a moment at the very beginning of the AIDS epidemic when a physician asked at an Infectious Disease Conference if AIDS might not be caused by a virus. His question was met with both irritation and annoyance by the members of the panel and the other physicians sitting in the audience.

This professional aversion to viruses is somewhat ingenuous

on the part of the medical community. It was only the discovery of antibiotics in the 1940s that kept physicians one step ahead of bacterial infections, and that step is getting smaller and smaller all the time. In 1956 there were over forty-eight different species of bacteria susceptible to the antibiotic tetracycline; in 1991 there were only three. Today there is only one antibiotic that can destroy the hospital-acquired infections caused by the coagulase-negative *Staphylococcus*. There is no antibiotic for patients infected with the gram-negative *Pseudomonas cepacia* bacillus. These patients simply die. There is a new effort on the part of the infectious disease establishment to develop bacteria-specific vaccines because in this age of growing antibiotic resistance, physicians realize they have no choice but to give the body its own chance to fight off bacterial invaders. Viruses never even offered physicians the chance to treat; was it little wonder, then, that viruses were viewed not only as mysterious but incomprehensible?

But some researchers and a few practitioners found viral diseases to be interesting and intriguing and, more importantly, refused to give up because no one was interested and the diseases were impossible to treat and difficult to study. These scientists, setting up their own agendas, used the electron microscope developed in the 1960s to work through the world of viruses as earlier scientists had used the light microscope to unravel the mysteries of bacteriology.

In short order virologists using the new microscope that magnified objects 200,000 times discovered in skin cells the rectangular particles that caused smallpox, the spherical particles in the brain cells of patients with measles and polio, the oblong particles in the saliva of rabid dogs, the tiny icosahedral hepatitis virus filling the liver cells of patients dying of yellow jaundice. But finding viral particles was one thing; initially, proving they caused disease proved to be quite another. At first no one could decide whether the particles found in diseased cells were alive or dead. At the time that viral particles were first seen, the accepted philosophical and scientific belief was that life, and therefore disease, was based on the cellular model of existence.

The finding of these tiny, solid, crystal-like structures, each less than one ten-thousandth the diameter of a cell, sitting in the cell's cytoplasm inert and unmoving like tiny lumps of coal, and then proposing these structures as the cause of some of man's most devastating diseases challenged accepted medical dogma and all of evolutionary theory.

The early virologists only compounded the controversy by being unable to grow these particles in cultures. But perhaps the most damaging argument against viruses causing disease was the fact that virologists never were able to find a single viral particle outside of a living cell or free of biological fluids. Unlike bacteria, molds, and fungi that were literally everywhere—in the air, on windowsills, near toilet seats, on vegetables, in the ground, and growing in showerheads—virus particles were only found in the cells of diseased and sick people. Indeed, under the electron microscope, these particles appeared totally inert. Yet, the virologists understood, these solid crystalline objects could and did cause disease. Pasteur's rabies agent passing through his porcelain filters was found to be viral particles. When virologists take a liver sample from an animal with hepatitis and grind up the tissues, pass the cellular components through a filter, collect the cell-free material below the filter, and then inject the filtrate into a healthy animal, they will find in the newly infected liver the same viral particles that were found in the liver of the original experimental animal.

The issue of exactly what viruses were and how they caused disease became even more confusing when experiments proved that while viruses *appeared* lifeless, they could still be killed. A filtrate from a liver of a patient with hepatitis or one from a brain of a patient with encephalitis, if exposed to alcohol or a few drops of Chlorox bleach and reinjected into a susceptible animal, would not cause disease, despite the fact that viral particles were clearly seen to be present in the injected filtrate.

And even more confusing, these inanimate particles appeared to be quite specific. The icosahedral virus that causes hepatitis only grows in liver cells and when injected only causes liver damage, the octagonal encephalitis virus only infects brain cells. Something else, too, became evident: namely, that viruses reproduce themselves and that they only produce more of themselves. A polio virus once inside a cell only produces another polio virus; a hepatitis virus only another hepatitis virus. Each apparently disease-causing virus only produces more of itself, or expressed more accurately, an exact replica of itself. There is clearly a kind of heredity, a quality only associated with life; and there is also a kind of intelligence, a knowing of where to go and how to get there, another basic characteristic of living things.

Virologists understood that in order to sort all this information out they had to do for viruses what Koch had done for bacteria: They had to find a way to grow viruses outside the body.

It was not to be an easy task. Since viruses only grew in cells, virologists had to learn how to grow cells so they could grow viruses. The researchers had to reconstitute what nature had evolved over a couple of billion years; but with perseverance and some good luck they first learned how to keep cells alive in Petri dishes and nutrient flasks and then how to get them to grow. They learned what amounts of oxygen cells needed to survive and what concentrations of trace elements; and they learned which antibiotics to add to the Petri dishes to keep bacteria from destroying the cell cultures and then which type of cells were necessary to grow which viruses. Just as Pasteur had injected his filterable agent into rabbits to develop his rabies vaccine, virologists took extracts of infected cells and used these extracts to infect their tissue cultures, continually transferring the viruses and, in the process, obtaining limitless amounts of pure virus samples. The ability to grow viruses turned a series of observations into a true science, well-organized and disciplined.

Virologists using their new supply of viruses quickly discovered that a virus particle was not as simple a structure as had first appeared. They found that viruses had an outer coat made of proteins but also had an inner core. They also found that when a viral particle came into contact with a susceptible cell, the particle actually stuck to the surface of that cell. After adhering to the cell for a very short time, less than a minute or two, the particle actually punctured the cell's outer wall and, mysteriously leaving its outer protein coat on the cell's surface, shot its inner core directly into the cell's cytoplasm. A chemical analysis of these inner cores showed that they were made up of strands of nucleic acids, but the strands of nucleic acids differed depending on the virus. Some viruses contained the conventional double helixes of DNA; others contained only a single strand of DNA, as if the virus contained only half the genetic code; and more confusing, a large number of viruses contained only strands of RNA. The discovery of strands of RNA and not DNA inside certain viruses was worrisome enough, but what confused everyone even more was that once these viral nucleotides were injected into a cell's cytoplasm, the virologists lost all track of them. The virologists couldn't find these nucleic acids anywhere; yet within a few hours to a few days, depending on the type of virus and the cell culture, new viral particles would mysteriously appear within the cell, each virus an exact replica of the original virus with an outside protein coat, inner core membrane, and the exact type of DNA or RNA that had been in the virus that had originally attached to the cell.

The accepted biological trinity of life, the one doctrine no scientist had questioned since Watson and Crick, was that DNA is transcribed into messenger RNA, the messenger RNA is then translated into proteins. And yet here in this new subcellular world of viruses, specifically of the viruses containing only RNA, the parts seemed to have turned around, and theory no longer fit the facts.

Still, the discovery that viruses had internal structures including particles of nucleic acids lead to two views on the origin of these particles. One view holds that viruses were once much more complicated cellular microorganisms that through a kind of backward evolution became less complicated and, in a way, more efficient. In this view, over time viruses slimmed themselves down to the barest essentials of reproduction, namely, an outer rigid protective core and an inner core containing replicating nucleotides that carry each virus's own specific genetic code.

The less dogmatic and more controversial view of viral evolution holds that viruses have always been the way they are—at the very borderlines of life—and that they simply never evolved much past the primeval soup stage of replicating polymers. In essence they have remained a kind of fossilized snapshot of the time when chemical evolution did indeed interface with the very beginnings of cellular life. In this view viruses as an evolutionary group simply took up residence in and around evolving cells and, never letting go, went along for the cellular evolutionary ride. It did not come as a surprise to some when the bacteriologists, using porcelain filters and tissue culture techniques, discovered that bacteria could become infected with viruses that they called "phage particles." What did come as a surprise was the discovery that these phage particles only infected bacteria and not animal cells and that infected bacteria actually produced enzymes, called "nucleases," that destroy the viruses by physically severing viral nucleotide sequences at certain points along the chain. It appears that during the struggle for survival, emerging bacteria developed the ability to defend themselves against viral attacks by producing enzymes that destroy the very essence of the ability of infecting viruses to divide and multiply. In the 1970s, it was discovered that the pneumococcal bacterium contains a nuclease that specifically severs adenine-thymine nucleotide linkages; the *Haemophilus influenzae* bacteria contain enzymes that cut cytosine-guanine linkages.

Researchers today use these bacterial nucleases to cut human DNA at specific points in order to map the different bases making up specific genes. But the discovery of the bacterial nucleases had another effect than the maps of nucleotide sequences; it gave virologists the clue they needed to discover how viruses cause cellular damage and, through that damage, disease. Virologists reasoned that bacteria's nucleases were produced to destroy the viral genes for a purpose. They understood that during a viral attack the virus injected its nucleic acids into the cell. The scientists assumed that the destruction eliminated the ability of those genes to take over the cell's machinery to make more viruses. Basically viruses cause disease by taking over the function of the cell's own genetic code, redirecting the cell's protein-making machinery to produce more viruses, the protein outer coat and inner cores and the enzymes the viruses need to survive and reproduce, stopping the cell from making the insulin or other hormones and proteins necessary for the whole organism to function, leading to cellular disease, tissue failure, and individual death.

A primitive yeast cell contains 100 genes that control all aspects of its life; a bacterium 3,000; the earthworm 20,000; and the mouse and human over 100,000. The increasing number of genes allows greater complexity as the genes code for more proteins. In the mouse over 200 different genes work together, each turning on and off at the correct time and in the proper sequence in order to form the brain, central nervous system, spinal cord, and connecting peripheral nerves, but if the blueprint changes, the necessary structural and neural transmitting proteins will be absent or altered and all the connections will fall apart, and the fetus will be born defective; in the case of humans, one child will be born with an abnormal brain, spinal bifida, or paralysis.

Today we know that those nucleotides the first virologists thought disappeared after a viral core is injected into a cell's cytoplasm never really vanish, and they do not stay out in the cell's cytoplasm. The injected viral genes do indeed go directly to the cell's nucleus, where they take over cellular control.

In the vast majority of viral infections, this incorporation lasts only a few hours, at the most a few days, before the body's immune system destroys the virus and cellular function returns to normal control. Those who view viruses as a stripped-down version of a cell set their moral judgments about disease aside and say that viruses simply have taken a more direct and chemically purer path to their own survival. There is no biological reason for a virus to carry its own cellular membranes, autocatalytic chemicals, endoplasmic reticula, and ribosomes to ensure its own existence if it can take over the cell's cytoplasmic machinery as its own. It is evolutionary predation at its most efficient. No need for scales or teeth—take over the software, become the new information system, and the world is yours.

The time scheme for viral diseases was considered to be virtually instantaneous until the 1970s when D. Carleton Gajdusek discovered what he called "slow viruses." Gajdusek felt that many of the neurologically degenerative diseases might be caused by "unconventional" viruses that induced disease years or, in most cases, decades after the cells became infected. He documented that kuru, a neurological disease first discovered in the tribes of New Guinea, was transmitted from person to person by cannibalism and that the eating of the infected brains of those killed in tribal warfare resulted in the disease's spreading among tribes and that the slow development of the disease virtually guaranteed the viruses continued transmission. Gajdusek showed that kuru could be transmitted experimentally to chimpanzees by inoculating them with homogenates of the brains of humans who had died of the disease, though it took years for the disease to develop in the inoculated monkeys.

Gajdusek's data were generally ignored and his theory that the majority of degenerative brain diseases might be caused by a transmissible agent that lay dormant in infected cells for thirty and forty years was just too much to consider—so this messenger, instead of being shot, was ignored, the message discarded. But Gajdusek proved to be only half right. Kuru and other human degenerative neurological diseases—including Creutzfeldt-Jakob, fatal familial insomnia, and Gerstmann-Sträussler-Scheinker disease as well as scrapie in sheep and bovine spongiform encephalopathy, or mad cow disease—are indeed caused by a transmissible infectious agent but not, as Gajdusek had thought, a virus.

It would take another thirty-five years before Gajdusek was proven wrong, but his idea of an infectious agent that lay dormant inside a cell for decades, if not the lifetime of the host, its genetic code hidden away without showing itself, yet remaining infectious would ensure a kind of virial survival quite different—and perhaps more efficient from an evolutionary standpoint—from an infection causing quick, irreversible cellular damage.

There are many infectious disease specialists today who, faced with the need to deal with a whole series of new viruses, resistant bacteria, and an increasing array of protozoan and fungal infections, have come to the conclusion that the battle may ultimately be unequal, that viruses, infectious agents, and microorganisms, having had an extra 2 billion years to get it right, aren't about to collapse or give up easily to any of the late arrivals.

Yet most people with viral illness recover. Smallpox disfigures, but in most cases it doesn't kill; only 5 percent of patients with measles end up with encephalitis; infectious mononucleosis is not a fatal disease; and not everyone with polio is crippled.

Human cells, unlike bacteria, do not contain nucleases, but we still are able to fight off viral infections. The question—and it is a fundamental one—is how do humans protect themselves from such attacks; how does the body know what to do; how does it know what is happening; how does it do what it has to do; or as the immunologist would say, "how do we know what is 'foreign' and what is 'self'?"

15

Disease is related to identity.

MOLECULAR GENETIC CONFERENCE

There exists in earthworms an early example of truly organized multicellular life—a primitive circulation—and in that circulation there exists an even more primitive cell. It is a cell so totally different from the creature's other cells that it looks as if it simply swam in one day and decided to stay. These independent, agile, ameboid cells, heavily armed with huge cytoplasmic granules, move through the tissue planes of the earthworm, working their way around and past the different cells, in and out of the circulatory channels, stopping here and there to pick up and digest bits and pieces of cellular debris like some kind of an efficient internal garbage system. What astonished the biologists who first saw these cells was that while they ingested fragmented membranes and decaying cellular proteins, they would, on occasion, pursue any bacteria that by design or chance had entered the body of the earthworm with the same aggressiveness with which they had attacked and ingested the bits of debris. These biologists, like all scientists, determined to name everything and anything, labeled these ameboid cells *phagocytes*, from the Greek word for "to ingest."

It became clear to a later generation of biologists that these phagocytes continued to exist in ever more sophisticated forms in the bloodstreams of all higher animals. Indeed, it is the offspring of these original ameboid cells that physicians measure today when they obtain a white count to see if a patient may be harboring an infection. The clear reason for maintaining a freely mobile independent cell as a part of evolution was the need for protection as an efficient circulatory system was gradually assembled.

The advantages of a circulatory system in a multicellular organism are obvious. The circulatory system becomes a stream that binds together the diverse tissues; it moves oxygen and nutrients from place to place; it removes waste products; it carries chemical signals from one group of cells to another; it allows for specialization within diversity and keeps all the parts working together. But evolution gives nothing away for free. There is a decided downside to an effective circulatory system.

The total blood volume in a human recirculates every thirteen seconds. A bacterium entering a cut finger can reach the lungs in under four seconds; a hepatitis virus in the colon can infect the liver in less than three; the meningococcus bacterium lodging in the nose or throat can reach the heart in under six seconds and move on to the brain or the sinus cavities in another five. Every cell of the body lies within the quick reach of the tides and drifts of the circulation. In the world of eat or be eaten, the advantages of a rapid and efficient circulatory system can quickly be turned against the organism. Multicellular organisms had to develop a rapid means of defense or the very circulation that allowed for increasing complexity, speed, and maneuverability would become the vehicle of their own destruction.

There was an argument among early embryologists as to whether phagocytes were in place before circulations evolved or whether the development of circulations pushed forward the rapid evolution of these carnivorous cells. Whichever did come first, once again the functions of protection and evolution were so interlaced that the inevitable conclusion must be that the body's phagocytes and its developing circulation existed and developed side by side, each evolving with ever-increasing sophistication as improvements in the other pushed them both forward. Today there are over a billion phagocytic cells at any one time moving through the circulation of most animals. The early phagocyte has evolved into three unique but clearly related groups of cells: the small mobile *neutrophil*, named for its nuclei that stain with neutral organic dyes; the more heavily armed *macrophage*, which contains hundreds of cytoplasmic granules, each containing over fifty different biologically active chemicals, all of which inhibit, immobilize, and kill bacteria; and the tissue *monocytes*, which lie in wait around veins and capillaries, ready to snatch up and destroy any passing microorganism. The importance of the early phagocytic cells and their modern-day descendants becomes painfully clear when one compares infections that occur in plants with those that affect animals.

The tobacco mosaic virus, crown gall disease, oak scorch, potato virus x, and fireblight are all diseases of plants caused by bacteria and viruses. While still deadly, these infections are for the most part localized and prolonged affairs. One leaf dies as another begins to grow; one part of a root system falters while another expands. The spread of disease and epidemics in plants proceeds in terms of weeks and months rather than seconds and minutes. An infection in a plant is, for the most part, a rather leisurely affair, but so is almost everything else about plant physiology. The movement of water and nutrients through a plant's tissues is a slow business. There are no rapid shifts here; no short-cuts for a microbe to spread rapidly from a root up to a leaf or branch, no infection one day and death the next. A diseased limb or abscessed trunk may eventually decay, but the rest of the plant lives on, giving up the infected part as it grows a new flower, even as the old flowers decay and die. It is not that microbes attacking plants are less destructive or less relentless than those that attack humans; they simply cannot spread as rapidly. But nature never relies on one system for anything as important as survival. Although time is on the side of plants, their tissues have also developed the ability to stop or at least control infections. In fact, plants turned the very slowness of their circulations to their advantage: Slowness was turned into a defense, holding immobilized bacterial and viral invaders in check while active chemicals produced in the leaf, stem, bark, or roots diffused into diseased areas to disable or kill the easily isolated intruder.

The stress of evolution put enormous biological pressure on plants to produce complicated molecules that, while slow to act, were quite effective if given enough time. It is this ability to produce very active chemical substances that we have exploited, an exploitation that once again shows the basic similarity of all life, for what works to protect plants from infections also works to protect our bodies from infections and diseases such as cancer. All the medicinal herbs and extracts, from digitalis to reserpine, paclitaxel, and vinblastine, as well as quinine, theophylline, and aspirin were first manufactured by plants to protect themselves from invading microbes. During evolution plants developed a rich and powerful store of biologically active molecules that acted as chemical defenses against predation by other cellular species. It is the fundamental nature of these structures and the chemical similarities of all living things that allow us to use quinine that the cinchona plant uses to stop a fungus to treat our malaria, the reserpine of the rauwolfia bush to control hypertension, while physicians use paclitaxel from the bark of the yew tree to destroy malignant ovarian cells.

But rapid circulations demanded a different strategy. The circulatory system had to carry its own defense; not only did it have to move its defenders around with speed and agility, it needed its defenses to be both nimble and overwhelming. There were to be no second chances.

In 1882, a Russian zoologist and trained microscopist, Elie Metchnikoff, on vacation in Messina, a town on Sicily's northeastern coast, pierced a tiny larva of the common starfish with a rose thorn. When he examined the larva twenty-four hours later, he saw tiny white cells surrounding the thorn, trying to destroy it. He understood immediately that these cells were trying to defend the larva by ingesting the invader. Within a year, Metchnikoff found these same cells in human circulation, noticing that during infections the number of these cells increased and stayed elevated until the infection subsided. Indeed, under the microscope, Metchnikoff was able to watch areas of infection and clearly saw how first the smaller, more mobile neutrophils entered the infected area, followed soon by the slower but more heavily armed macrophages. He watched how the macrophages and neutrophils ingested the bacteria and how, once inside the cell, the bacteria were destroyed.

Physicians in the sixteenth, seventeenth, and eighteenth centuries had debated the issue of what was called "good pus versus bad pus." Pus that was thick and dark was viewed as a warning that the patient was not improving; a thinner, watery pus, somewhat blood-tinged, particularly after a period of heavier pus production, was viewed as a sign that the patient was improving. It was a desperate and crazy distinction, like smelling urine to diagnose kidney or bladder stones, but at least it had the virtue of making physicians touch and examine their patients.

Metchnikoff clarified the whole issue of pus, "good" and "bad," by proving that the material was in reality a mixture of billions of dead and dying bacteria that had been fighting it out with billions of attacking neutrophils and macrophages; the type of pus depended on both the species of invading bacteria and, strangely, whatever was the most prominent type of phagocyte—neutrophil or macrophage.

Metchnikoff's microscope showed that there was no subtlety in this fight, no death at a distance here, no smart bombs or standoff weapons. The body's lighter, more mobile neutrophils and the larger, more heavily granulated macrophages slugged it out with bacteria, cell to cell, and cytoplasm to cytoplasm. Pus, whether squeezed from a pimple or drained from a hepatic abscess, is the visible—if microscopic—manifestation of what has become nature's means of granting success or failure.

Metchnikoff felt that in his observations of phagocytes he had discovered how the body fights infections. He presented such dramatic evidence and so warlike a picture that most physicians became convinced that neutrophils and macrophages were not only one of the means by which a body protects itself against infection but, indeed, the only way it defends itself. If Metchnikoff wondered how his famous phagocytes knew where to go or how they actually managed to kill the bacteria and, of course, why they never attacked the body's own tissues, he never mentioned it; he was content, it seems, with his theory just as it was.

But other scientists did wonder and made their own discoveries that did not quite fit with the simple "stimulate the phagocyte" scenario of defense. It was discovered in the laboratories of England and Germany that when a person becomes infected with bacteria, there suddenly appears in that person's bloodstream a protein that, when purified and mixed with a culture of the infecting bacteria, causes the bacteria to clump together. There was clearly more going on during infections than the marshaling up of a flood of attacking phagocytes.

Working in Germany, Emil von Behring, showed that when a person is infected with the diphtheria bacillus, the person produces a very specific protein that enters the circulation and actually neutralizes the toxin produced by the infecting bacillus. Behring called this neutralizing substance "antitoxin" and, purifying the material, went on to show that the symptoms of diphtheria, the swollen neck, difficulty breathing, heart and kidney failure, could all be prevented by injecting his purified antitoxin into the bloodstream after a person was infected. Behring made it clear that his diphtheria antitoxin had nothing at all to do with Metchnikoff's granulocytes, but he could not explain how or where the antitoxin was produced.

Koch, too, had found some unexpected results during his own pursuit of bacterial infections. During a series of classic experiments he injected tuberculin, a substance extracted from the cell walls of the tuberculosis bacillus, into guinea pigs already infected with the disease. If the extract was injected into the guinea pig's skin, a terrible reaction occurred, leading to ulcers and deep scars. Koch and his colleagues examined the scarred skin and found to their amazement that the damaged tissue was filled not with Metchnikoff's phagocytes but with other rather benign-looking cells called "lymphocytes." These small, round cells, mostly all nucleus with only a slight rim of cytoplasm, contained absolutely no granules but circulated along with the phagocytes. Metchnikoff had even drawn these small, passive, benign-looking cells with their modest supply of clear cytoplasm in his scientific diagrams, sitting there in the circulation next to the highly mobile neutrophils and more heavily armed macrophages. Earlier anatomists had also noticed these small cells, not in the bloodstream but in the body's lymph nodes, so they were given the name *lymphocytes*. Hematologists, too, had found these same cells in bone marrow, but the cells looked so inactive, so passive, that they were ignored and discussed, if at all, almost as an afterthought. Yet, as Koch would write, these cells had somehow worked their way into the areas of his tuberculin injections and were clearly part of a terrible skin reaction.

But Koch's tuberculin story didn't end with the skin. If Koch injected his tuberculin extract directly into the bloodstream of an already infected guinea pig, the animal's lungs quickly filled with fluid, the heart would dilate and the animal, convulsing with seizures, would be dead within seconds. A live tuberculin bacillus was not injected, yet something catastrophic had occurred by simply injecting a part of the bacterium's cell wall. There appeared to be more to the dangers of infection than just the invasion of a live microbe, something quite a bit older and perhaps even more basic.

Charles Robert Richet, working in America in the 1920s, proved that even if something innocuous as the white of an egg were injected into an animal's bloodstream, followed by a second injection a week or two later, the animals like Koch's guinea pigs would be dead within minutes after the second injection. Richet wondered if there was not some connection between the disastrous results following the injection of tuberculin into a previously infected guinea pig and his repeated injection of egg white into an animal already exposed to the same protein.

During the years that Behring was trying to characterize his diphtheria antitoxin, Koch and Richet were injecting their extracts. A colleague of Behring, Richard Pfeiffer, showed just how basic and interrelated all these experiments actually were. He injected bacteria directly into the bloodstream of animals previously infected with the same bacteria and made the discovery that the bacteria, once injected, not only clumped together, but a number were immediately destroyed within the animal's circulation by what Pfeiffer called "serum factors." Indeed, Pfeiffer never saw a single granulocyte in or near any of these dying bacteria. He actually watched as the bacteria, once in the animal's bloodstream, simply swelled up, and then, as if suddenly dynamited, actually exploded into hundreds of tiny pieces.

It did not come as a surprise to these "serum factor" scientists when it was discovered that the primitive circulations of worms, lampreys, and hagfish—animals that had remained virtually unchanged for over 600 million years—also contained this ability to detonate invading bacteria.

By the early 1930s, the scientists who studied how the body defends itself had divided themselves into two camps. One group, the Metchnikoff clique, was convinced that defense resided solely in the granulocytes; the other, the Behring group, proposed that the real answer to how the body defends itself lay in serum factors that were produced during or after exposure to "foreign substances," by what they called the body's "humoral" or "antibody system."

A German biologist finally proved what no one had suspected or even considered—that everyone was right. Protection against invading microorganisms is simply too important to be left to any one system. So important is the need to be able to defend against the microscopic world of infectious agents that evolution had devised two systems of defense. The first, the phagocyte system, is made up of the body's white cells, its neutrophils, macrophages, and monocytes; the second, the immune system, is made up of its own two parts: the humoral system, composed of antibodies and antitoxins, and the cellular, made up of the body's lymph nodes and its circulating lymphocytes. When in the early 1940s it was discovered that the body's white cells are better able to destroy bacteria coated with antibodies produced by the humoral system, it seemed that there was really only one defense system, all the parts working together and—in a very real and fundamental way—talking to each other in a chemical conversation that began more than 3 billion years ago, a conversation that over the millennia a number of bacteria and viruses, including the AIDS virus, have learned to frustrate and then disrupt.

16

People react to fear, not love.
They don't teach that in Sunday School.

RICHARD M. NIXON

In the early days of AIDS, when the prevalence of the disease among homosexuals led physicians to give the epidemic the acronym GRID for gay related immune deficiency, there were a few who understood that it was not only gays who would suffer. In the spring of 1983 an African physician wrote to a colleague in Europe, "This is going to be a world class disaster." But it was the British physicians at the London School of Tropical Medicine who had the first clear, if brutal, insight into what had happened. The British, with their fabled restraint, postulated an intraspecies transfer of a virus as the cause of AIDS.

Dr. J. Seale wrote in the *Journal of the Royal Society of Medicine* that a transfer of viruses across species lines had been reported before, but such a transfer had usually been restricted in scope. Ebola hemorrhagic fever, Marburg disease, Lassa and Rift Valley fevers were all viral infections that had been discovered to occur normally only in rodents and monkeys but when transferred to humans, presumably through inhalation or bites, caused infections that were inevitably fatal and, as Seale wrote, ". . . so quickly fatal that there is no ability to maintain an epidemic." But it hardly benefits an infecting bacterium or virus to kill its host. A perfect world to a microbe such as the *Helicobacter pylori* bacillus would be to infect a person and then live untouched in its own environmental niche, safe and secure with time to divide, grow, and multiply. Death simply does not benefit a parasite or its host. Indeed, for obvious reasons most infections reach a kind of equilibrium with their victims. Many biologists have talked about the relationship between an infecting agent and its host. It is a balance; in a very real way it depends on the personality of the agent and the extent to which the agent and the host share their own agendas for survival. They may agree to get along: The host reproduces and stays relatively healthy or healthy for long periods of time and the attacker or, in the case of viruses, its genes go along for the ride. But it can go the other way, as the relationship between the rabies virus and its host cells so clearly illustrates. The virus has no interest in its host's survival. There is no shared agenda . . . get inside the cells, rob the bank, and get away in the saliva to attack another animal. Seale merely pointed out the obvious. The monkeys and rodents infected with viruses fatal to humans appear to do quite well. Presumably the animals originally infected that were unable to defend themselves had over the centuries died off, while the immune systems of the surviving animals had worked out a deal with these same viruses—they would live together, each keeping the other more or less intact. Still, Seale reasoned, if such an intraspecies transfer did not quickly kill the infected person, or if a transferred virus had a long incubation period, the result of such a cross-species transfer would produce a self-sustaining epidemic or "a lethal pandemic of a magnitude unparalleled in human history." There was no discussion here of correct sexual practices, God's punishment, or personal retribution. Seale merely stated a biological fact.

Seale's view of viruses crossing species, with initial disastrous results for their new hosts, became all too real, and not in Africa but in the state of New Mexico. A 1994 article in *New England Journal of Medicine* paraphrased the more pragmatic Seale:

> On May 14, 1993, the New Mexico office of the medical investigator was notified of the unexplained deaths of a couple living in the same household in rural New Mexico: a 21-year-old woman and a 19-year-old man. Both died of acute respiratory failure—the man within five days after the woman. By May 17, Indian Health Service physicians had reported five deaths from adult respiratory distress syndrome among previously healthy adults. . . . results of laboratory studies of serum and tissue samples from several patients suggested an acute infection with a new species of Hantavirus. . . . an immuno-histochemical analysis revealed widespread endothelial [blood vessel] distribution of viral antigen in the lungs, kidneys, heart, pancreas, adrenal glands and skeletal muscle cells. . . . The Hantaviruses have now been isolated from several species of rodents found in both rural and urban settings in the United States.

A number of infectious disease experts, growing more and more concerned about the emergence and spread of cross-species viral infections, are pursuing these outbreaks with some success. What is evident from their studies is that apparently novel viruses are in reality viruses that have existed for hundreds of thousands, if not millions of years. They are only now becoming evident because of the growth of human populations into once inaccessible areas of great biodiversity and the rapid movement of humans from place to place.

The Ebola virus kills so quickly that it truly leaves no tracks. Scientists have tried to find its host, literally testing all living things along the Ebola River basin. The researchers have found nothing, but in comparing the virus's gene sequences coding for surface markers, they found that the virus in its different outbreaks, separated by as long as twenty years, are exact matches. This lack of significant mutation has led virologists to believe that the Ebola virus has remained in a very stable niche for quite some time and that whatever host harbors the virus, that animal does not migrate. Nor has the virus changed between outbreaks.

But in the early 1980s, the majority of scientists were not concerned about cross-species infections, and the rest wanted to forget what was already known. In fact, it was only the original clustering of AIDS among homosexuals and hemophiliacs that alerted physicians to the fact that something new and terrible and unexpected had invaded the human race.

It has always been the clusterings of infectious disease in certain areas, or in specific groups, that alerted physicians to the infectious rather than inherited or congenital nature of disease. The rubella virus has always infected humans, but it took the grouping of large numbers of working women in the factories of World War II, some of whom were pregnant, for public health officials to realize that the development of a specific type of congeni-tal defect, including the combination of heart disease, blindness, and large spleens, was not simply bad luck for the developing child or the exposure of the mother to environmental toxins but the result of an infection with the rubella virus. These congenital defects were the result of pregnant women being infected in their first trimester with what had been considered to be a benign virus, but which, in reality, had the ability to cross the placenta and infected developing fetuses. Because of the grouping of these congenital defects in the infants of factory workers, physicians were able to work backward and find that all the women giving birth to these malformed infants had experienced the rash and other symptoms of German measles, establishing the fact that the rubella virus was the cause of these congenital defects.

Recently it was the clustering of pneumonias in thirty-four American Legionnaires having their state convention in the same hotel that alerted infectious disease specialists that there was a unique bacterium growing in the hotel's air conditioning system and spreading through the air vents that was infecting humans, causing pneumonias and death. What was important about the discovery of Legionnaire's disease was not that a new, dangerous bacterium had been discovered but that those earlier cases of people dying from pneumonias after staying in hotels were not due to smoking or fate but exposure to a bacterium that, if treated early enough with the correct antibiotic, could be cured.

In reality, that early clustering of disease and death among homosexuals and hemophiliacs gave the research community a five-year head start on discovering the cause of AIDS. It was the true sacrifice of these two groups that saved the rest of us from the fate of the villagers of central Africa and our children the short, miserable lives of the thousands of Romanian infants exposed to HIV-contaminated blood.

As a society, we barely dodged a bullet. In truth, it was only the scientists involved in studies of infectious disease, virology, molecular biology, genetics, and immunology who allowed us to work out what was really happening and, in the process, they gave each of us the ability to save ourselves and our loved ones. But like so many of those paradoxes of human success, the new understandings of how we defend ourselves came out of our baser motives . . . specifically, the perceived need to kill each other.

17

In any great mystery, there is always a mastermind.

MYSTERY WRITERS SEMINAR

The naval battles of World War II, particularly along the cargo routes of the North Atlantic, led to a new kind of trauma patient, a patient for whom the medical profession as well as medical science was ill-prepared. Between 1940 and 1943 the number of British sailors burned when their ships were torpedoed had increased to such an extent that special hospital units throughout the British Isles had to be set aside as burn wards. The outcome for these burn patients was grim. Patients with third-degree burns over more than 60 percent of their bodies did not survive longer than two weeks. If the patients didn't die of massive fluid loss, they died of overwhelming infection as bacteria colonized their charred skin and then worked their way down into the patient's circulation and deeper tissues. It was clear to physicians that the burned skin had to be replaced both to protect from fluid loss and to protect against infection.

Peter Medawar, a biology professor at Oxford, was asked by the British government to look at skin grafting as a possible treatment for these patients. Skin grafts had been tried on burn

patients before but never in a very organized or scientific manner; and more importantly, when grafts had been tried they inevitably failed. Medawar was too good a scientist not to know
that he needed an experimental model to control the variables of
skin grafting and give him the ability to sort out the reasons for
these failures. Medawar chose for his studies the most common
laboratory animal—the mouse.

Medawar began his experiments by covering burned areas of
experimental mice with mouse skin. Even when the grafts were
sutured into place, he found that after a few days they would
begin to come loose, shrivel up, and eventually fall off, but not,
as he had expected, from infections but rather from an invasion
of the graft by thousands of the recipient mouse's own lymphocytes. It seemed to be Koch's tuberculin story all over again.
Thousands of lymphocytes had somehow left the mouse's bloodstream and invaded the graft, first destroying the attachments of
the graft to the normal skin and then continuing on until the
whole graft was consumed.

The unexpected presence of such large numbers of lymphocytes in the grafts surprised Medawar. Despite the tuberculin
studies, lymphocytes were considered to be inactive cells, mere
bystanders in the fight for survival. Those who supported the
phagocytic theory of immune protection, as well as those who
championed the humoral view of immunity, had ignored these
strange little cells for so long that it came as a shock to
Medawar and his associates to see them in huge numbers invading a donor graft.

Putting aside his surprise, Medawar continued his studies, re-
fining as he went along. He proved that no matter what the degree of burn, the area burned, or the size or depth of the burn,
there was always a precise, reproducible series of cellular events
that began within an hour of a graft being put in place. These
events continued in a clearly reproducible manner until the graft
was destroyed. The scenario was always the same. At first a few

of the mouse's neutrophils entered the edges of the graft and then quickly withdrew. Over the next few hours, a small number of lymphocytes began to arrive. Between twelve and twenty-four hours, additional lymphocytes started to flood into the graft from all directions, new ones arriving virtually every minute, the mass of cells working their way deeper and deeper into the graft. Eventually, completely infiltrated by lymphocytes, the graft began to die and eventually it fell off. Later researchers were to find this same sequence of events occurring in the rejection of transplanted organs.

But in 1944, Medawar had to reach beyond himself and become a magician. He began his skin graft experiments all over again, only this time he used genetically identical mice. The grafts did not fall off; there were no invading lymphocytes; the skin grafts thrived. Medawar then began a series of genetically graded experiments using mice that were related but with different degrees of genetic closeness. He quickly showed that the severity and degree of graft destruction depended on the genetic relationship between the donor mouse and the recipient. Medawar proved that no matter what the degree, size, or depth of the burn, grafts exchanged between genetically identical mice were never rejected and that in genetically dissimilar mice the severity of the rejection increased as the genetic diversity increased.

Medawar understood that his experiments proved more than the fact that genetics played a role in donor graft rejections; they showed for the first time that heredity and, therefore, genes were fundamental to the whole affair and that the genes involved in rejection worked their magic through the seemingly passive lymphocytes.

Advances in science are carried forward on the backs of magicians and geniuses, and, since science is a measuring discipline, on new technologies that measure new dimensions. Galileo needed his telescope before Kepler could establish his Laws of

Planetary Motions. The study of Medawar's lymphocytes was carried forward by a Swedish biochemist, Arne Tiselius, who developed an instrument that separated proteins on the basis of their overall electrical charge, not on the old bases of molecular weights, freezing or melting points, or resistance to solvents. Tiselius discovered that the different number of carbon, nitrogen, and hydrogen atoms that make up amino acids gave each its own unique electrical charge. When combined in a protein, each charge adds together to give each protein a unique overall electrical fingerprint. Tiselius's machine was able to make very fine separations of proteins. The machine contained a neutral gel that allowed proteins to move through a constant electrical charge. Proteins placed in the gel migrated at different speeds, the more negatively charged proteins moving faster toward the positive pole than the less-charged molecules. The development of this electrophoresis machine exploited the physical differences in the charge of proteins to first separate and then examine pure samples of these molecules. The electrophoresis machines established that three different classes of proteins exist in the human circulations: the *alpha globulins*, the *beta globulins*, and the *gamma globulins*.

In the early 1940s two infants were admitted to the pediatric ward of Walter Reed Army Hospital. The hospital's pathology department was routinely using an electrophoresis machine to test the serum of patients for a control study to develop replacement plasma products for wounded soldiers. The children had been admitted for recurrent upper respiratory and ear infections, failure to thrive, and repeated fungal infections of their mouths and throats, and—more ominous—an increasing number of severe pneumonias. By mistake, their blood was drawn and tested. Physicians going over the data were astonished to find that these children had absolutely no gamma globulins in their blood.

The discovery that serum of children with severe, recurrent infections did not contain any gamma globulins focused the attention of the world's medical community on the importance of the gamma globulin fraction of blood in fighting infections. It was quickly discovered that all antibodies, from Behring's antitoxins to Pfeiffer's serum factors, were themselves gamma globulins. The discovery that antibodies were gamma globulins and that children without the ability to make gamma globulins were susceptible to infections forced the physicians to recheck the children's blood. The number of lymphocytes in their circulation were also markedly reduced. During his experiments Medawar had found traces of gamma globulins along with the lymphocytes in the rejected skin grafts, but he did not understand the significance of his discovery.

In 1960 Medawar received the Nobel Prize for his rejection studies, but by that time his graft experiments, along with the electrophoresis studies on gamma globulins, had a host of researchers focusing their attention on the once ignored and cast-off lymphocyte.

18

*There is more to fighting battles
than merely documenting the warriors.*

ANONYMOUS

We have each felt the small glands in our neck that swell up when we have a sore throat or develop tonsillitis. The Greeks and Romans noticed them too, as did medieval physicians; in fact, virtually every generation of healers has remarked how nodes in the groin swell when legs are infected and the nodes in the arm increase in size with a wound of the hand. These glands were described by the earliest anatomists and battlefield surgeons as being present not only in the neck, arm, and groin but literally and figuratively everywhere in the body. There was not a tissue, organ, or major blood vessel that did not have a number of these nodes either surrounding it or, at least, close by. Physicians explained that these glands acted as filters, straining out evil humors and, when microbiology came into vogue, trapping and killing bacteria. Eighteenth- and nineteenth-century physicians maintained this fiction despite the fact that no bacteria were ever found within a swollen lymph node. All that was ever found within an enlarged node was an increased number of lymphocytes.

It was observed by early clinicians that lymph nodes nearest a cut or inflamed area were the nodes that increased in size; nodes further away from the damaged site remained quite unchanged. What was surprising in Medawar's rejection studies was that the lymph nodes closest to the grafts were also noticed to have increased in size.

There was clearly a relationship among lymph nodes, lymphocytes, and the organism's ability to fight infections or reject skin grafts. The problem was that no one could find a system.

It was easy to find a cardiovascular system; there were a heart, arteries, veins, and connecting capillaries. The digestive system was clearly made up of the mouth, esophagus, stomach, and small and large intestine; everyone could see that the nervous system consisted of the brain, spinal cord, and peripheral nerves. The connections between the parts are obvious, the notion of a system self-evident.

But where was the immune system? The effectiveness of vaccines, the rejection of skin grafts, and the production of antibodies, the elimination of viral infections, and the destruction of bacteria all indicated some kind of well-ordered, precise, interactive system, but where and how? If the biological dogma that structure begets function is correct, where are the structures that make the antibodies to fight infections and reject skin grafts, while ordering the precise release of the body's neutrophils, macrophages, and lymphocytes.

In the 1960s, Robert Coleman, an immunologist focusing on lymphocytes, found a way to remove these cells from the bloodstream and label them with a tiny radioactive label. He then injected the labeled lymphocytes back into circulation and used new scanning devices to monitor their movements through the body. He found that the labeled lymphocytes did not just float around inside the circulation, indiscriminately drifting here and there; rather, each followed well-organized and defined routes. Without any apparent means of locomotion, these cells moved quickly through the blood vessels, into the capillaries, and then out into the tissues and organs of the body and then back to the nearest lymph node. The lymphocytes then moved through the lymph nodes and once again went back into the circulation, to begin another virtually identical circuit through the body. Coleman learned not only that circulating lymphocytes picked their own unique paths through the body but that these vagabond lymphocytes appeared to live forever, moving in and out of the tissues and through the body's lymph nodes in a regular, predictable fashion for the life of the person.

All lymphocytes looked alike under the microscope, but a more detailed biochemical and structural analysis showed that there were in reality two distinctly different types of lymphocytes, with completely different biological abilities and immunological functions. During fetal development the cells that are eventually to evolve into adult lymphocytes go through their own individual transformations. Embryologists, following the maturation of lymphocytes from their production by cells in fetal bones, discovered that these immature lymphocytes went literally in one of two directions. The cells either left the bone marrow and went to the developing stomach or went to a gland in the fetal neck called the thymus. The lymphocytes that reached these fetal glands were exposed to different signal proteins produced by the tissues of each gland that activate specific genes in the immature lymphocytes so that when the cells leave these glands, each type of lymphocyte has such different abilities that the embryologists could clearly tell the differences and were able to give the cells two different names. The cells leaving the stomach were called B lymphocytes, cells able to produce antibodies; those that left the thymus were the body's T lymphocytes, cells that do not make antibodies but can attack and destroy individual bacteria, parasites, and virally infected cells, as well as transplanted foreign tissues.

Scientists finally realized that over its long history the body's immune system learned to tailor its response to the type of attacker and they learned where specifically those attackers infect the body. The majority of bacteria and parasitic worms infect the bloodstream, tissue fluids, and the intestinal tract. The immune system uses its B lymphocytes to make the water-soluble antibody proteins that move through the body's fluids and bind directly to the surfaces of these extracellular organisms.

Viruses, the tuberculosis bacillus, and a number of intracellular microbes, such as malaria and *Pneumocystis carinii* protozoa, that directly infect cells and are not easily reached by antibodies are attacked by T lymphocytes, which are able to produce an astonishing number of chemicals and enzymes, called "mediators" and "cytokines," that diffuse out of the T cell's cytoplasm into infected cells. It is these chemical mediators that suppress viral replication or damage and kill the intracellular parasites. These mediators can also impede the division of abnormal cells while attracting more T cells and other neutrophils into the battle area. The cytokines are so biologically active and chemically powerful that they can destroy malignant cells. Some of these T-lymphocyte cells become so relentless in their attacks and so determined to destroy anything found to be "nonself," that the immunologists have given them the name *killer T cells*.

Immunologists studying lymphocytes in the test tube found they were able to distinguish the two types of lymphocytes not only by their function but by various unique surface proteins, or markers, embedded in their outer cell membranes.

At the very beginnings of biological evolution, genes coded early for the construction of proteins making up cellular walls. In the shift over from single-cell to multicellular life, organisms derived from single cells sharing the same cell wall structures had an obvious advantage over creatures composed of cells with different types of walls. Economy needs order, and under the increasing pressures of complexity and competition where functions had to be shared, the ability to tell what fit and what belonged, what would always be present, what could be counted on to help, and what was reliable had a clear advantage and thus value over what might or might not work, what might or might not be there, or what might simply be a visitor or, worse, an inadequate imposter. Identical surface structures became part of existence, a means for the different assembly of parts to tell from the very beginnings of multicellular life what was self and what was a stranger. The prescription for multicellular creatures that eventually won the race of evolution was the single dividing cell, carrying its single set of chromosomes forward into each new cell so that tissues not only share abilities but the same surfaces and with those abilities and surfaces, the same identity and the same history. Genetic identification spelled out through shared surface structures became both the means of identity and a protective force in an ever more competitive world.

In the 1930s, it was discovered that genes on chromosome 17 in mice and a similar series of genes in humans on chromosome 6, labeled by immunologists the major histocompatibility complex (given the abbreviation MHC), produce two types of proteins, the class I and class II molecules that are assembled at the cell's surface, where they become part of the cell membrane. So important are these surface markers that every human cell has between half a million and a million class I molecules on each surface.

Since every fertilized egg has its own unique genetic code, each cell of an individual will carry that same code and will have precisely the same array of proteins and markers present on its surfaces. The human MHC complex contains over 100 genes made up of over 4 million base pairs, leading to the possibility of over a trillion different markers.

All cells of an individual share the same class I markers, and it is these molecules that are used for recognition. There is little chance for "molecular mimicry" here. You either belong or you don't.

The body's T cells, macrophages, and neutrophils carry the additional class II surface markers. These proteins are not only used for identification among the diverse cells of the immune system; they are also used by those cells to exchange bits of foreign surfaces scavenged from attacking bacteria and viruses as information, which the cells of the immune system carry back to the lymph nodes to activate killer T cells and tell the B cells which antibodies to make. Some of the mystery of how the body fights infection was settled when it was discovered that when a virus invades a cell, the cell wall changes as parts of the virus's inner cores are carried to the cell's surface, transforming it so that the circulating immune cells can read the surface as foreign.

The rest of the mystery was settled in the middle 1970s, when two researchers working in Australia performed a series of experiments that proved T lymphocytes recognized virally infected cells only in the wider context of class I and class II molecules. The experiments were deceptively simple; the researchers, like Medawar before them, used different strains of infected mice. The scientists discovered that T lymphocytes were indeed capable of killing a virus-infected cell, but only if the virally infected cell was from the same strain of mice as the injected lymphocytes. It was clear that not only do viral particles have to be physically presented on the surfaces of infected cells, but both the infected cell and the attacking T lymphocytes have to share identical surface markers. The cells of the immune system will make the fight, but only for their own kind.

In what is clearly an example of phase-shifting, it was found that the white cells also use their surface markers as homing receptors to hook onto proteins making up the cell surfaces of blood vessel walls so they can work their way out of the circulation into areas of infection. It became clear that during evolution the proteins making up cell surfaces took on more functions than those of structural integrity identification and transfer of information about infection and invaders. A molecule of insulin released by a cell in the pancreas binds to an insulin receptor site on the surface of a muscle cell, which permits that muscle cell to remove sugar from the circulation and use that sugar as an energy source allowing it to contract. What was once simply a surface structure has become a receptor allowing the two cells, the insulin producer and the contracting muscle cell, even though separated, to talk to each other.

Another part of the puzzle surrounding immunity fell into place after a series of recurring blunders occurred when thoracic surgery was getting its start. Occasionally during a chest operation a surgeon would inadvertently sever a tiny, thin-walled structure near the heart. The chest would immediately fill with a thick, milky fluid, which was found under a microscope to contain millions of lymphocytes. In every generation anatomists had described a similar series of thin-walled channels running throughout the body, but the channels were so delicate and so easily destroyed during dissections that their paths were impossible to follow for more than a few millimeters.

These thin-walled channels were not arteries or veins but the body's third great highway system. The duct that the thoracic surgeons cut was the final pathway of the system allowing the body's circulating lymphocytes to reach the heart, to be pumped back out in the body to begin their travels through the tissues and lymph nodes in their never-ending circuits.

Nature had surprised everybody. There was indeed no single, well-defined immune system. Protection was too important to be left in any one place, so nature had placed it everywhere and kept it moving.

19

States are made up of a considerable number of the ignorant and foolish, a small proportion of genuine knaves, and a sprinkling of capable and honest men, by whose efforts the former are kept in a reasonable state of ignorance and the latter of repression.

THOMAS HUXLEY

When the first AIDS antibody test became available, serum samples that had been stored in the freezers of the clinics and hospitals across central Africa were examined for the presence of the antibody to the virus. The reason for this evaluation was the logical assumption that the earliest presence of an antibody specific for the virus would indicate, at least approximately, the date of the beginning of the epidemic. As a science, immunology has reached such precision that researchers were confident that the body's immune system would be a better detector of a new virus entering the human population than any of their own epidemiological studies. No antibodies were found before 1968. There were a few positive blood samples in early 1970, the numbers increasing through the 1970s, and then doubling and quadrupling with every additional year.

Physicians at the Institute for Tropical Diseases in England now consider the European AIDS epidemic to have occurred in two waves. They considered the first phase, beginning in the early 1970s, to be the result of the transfer of the virus from central Africa to Europe. The second and much larger epidemic, beginning in the early 1980s, resulted from the virus being carried back into the major cities of France, England, Germany, and Italy from the cities of North America.

In 1982 the Congressional Research Service compiled the mortality rates on AIDS and, forced by their own data to scrap the inappropriate and misleading acronym GRID, designated the disease AIDS, for acquired immune deficiency syndrome, to distinguish it from the condition of those few infants born without any immune system. The 1982 report was ominously prophetic. Forty percent of those patients diagnosed in the late 1970s were dead; the mortality among AIDS patients had reached 60 percent within five years of infection. More ominous still, the rate of new cases had tripled in the first two years of the decade and the data showed that the increase would continue. There were so many new patients that the sheer mass of routine laboratory work was making some laboratory observations almost impossible—but the clinical results were obvious and distressing. Physicians were simply surprised by how sick and miserable these patients were. All had severe diarrhea; all had terrible, painful sores in their mouths that kept them from eating and drinking; all soon became dehydrated; most were in some kind of pain; all had high fevers; all had large, swollen lymph nodes; most eventually developed severe pneumonias; all were confused; many had seizures; the majority were anemic; and some were in heart failure.

The report on AIDS was distributed at approximately the same time that eight people mysteriously died from what was discovered to be the tampering with Tylenol capsules by adding cyanide. These poisonings were front-page news for weeks; the government mobilized its forces; the manufacturer of Tylenol pulled its product off the shelves of every drugstore in the United States, while shipments of Tylenol being sent to Canada and Mexico were stopped at the borders. Eight deaths had mobilized the country; and yet with the ever-increasing incidence of AIDS, with dozens of hemophiliacs dying from pneumocystis lung infections, the numbers of infants born with AIDS doubling every year, our nation's drug industry, our politicians, public health officials, and the administrators of blood banks denied that anything was wrong.

An executive of the blood bank industry announced at the beginning of 1983 that there was no need for testing the U.S. blood supply, that "the risk of getting AIDS from a transfusion is about one in a million." The medical establishment rallied in support of its blood banks, refusing to insist on any restrictions on blood donors. Dr. Joseph Bore, the chairman of the American Association of Blood Banks, stated that "even if, and it's still a big if, a small number of AIDS cases turn out to be transfusion-related, I do not believe that this can be interpreted to mean that our blood supply is contaminated." At the same time that Bore was making his self-serving statement, events were proving the opposite in the cities of North America. Randy Shilts, the author of *And the Band Played On*, a chronology of the AIDS epidemic, revealed the duplicity of corporate and public officials all through the early 1980s:

In Los Angeles, a thirty-eight-year-old nurse who had received a blood transfusion during a hysterectomy was ailing from pneumocystis. Her condition had been watched anxiously by Los Angeles health officials ever since one of the donors for her November 1982 transfusion answered affirmatively to question 44 of the questionnaire given to all local AIDS patients: "Have you ever been a blood or plasma donor in the last five years."

Within two weeks of the transfusion, the nurse was suffering from lymphadenopathy.

Yet at the same time Adrian Killner, M.D., of the New York Blood Center wrote, "We're not convinced that AIDS is transmitted by blood transfusions . . . the evidence is very shaky."

In the middle 1990s, it was discovered that executives of the blood supply industry consciously released pools of high-risk serums specifically obtained from young homosexual males as a potential treatment for patients with hepatitis B into the general blood product distribution system.

In September of 1984, the Centers for Disease Control documented eighty new cases of transfusion AIDS, a quadrupling of confirmed cases from the year before. In November of that year the first case of placentally transferred AIDS from a pregnant mother with hemophilia to her newborn child was clearly documented. That same year a Roman Catholic nun died from a blood transfusion given during a hip replacement operation performed in July of 1982. At the funeral mass, the priest explained during the homily that the nun had spent her final days praying for the person who had donated the infected blood. Even early in the epidemic, those afflicted, including priests and nuns, knew the commercial blood supply of the country was contaminated, while those in charge continued to deny that there was anything wrong.

The original perception of AIDS as a homosexual disease may have made a public health attack on the disease politically incorrect, but it was the sheer desire for profit that kept blood banks officials and their employed physicians from removing contaminated blood from the distribution system. It has yet to end.

In January of 1994, the German press acknowledged:

The government health agency has hushed up a six-year-old suspicion that hundreds of patients received AIDS-tainted blood during transfusions. . . . Health Minister Horst Sechofer has announced that the pharmaceutical company was allowed to use a cheaper, less-sensitive screening test for AIDS, allowing tainted blood into the system.

Snow had only his maps and his own personal conviction to convince the people of London that it was their water that was killing their wives and children. By the end of 1984, no one needed a map to convince politicians or physicians that AIDS was a sexually transmittable viral disease and that the virus had entered the world's blood supply.

But the perception of the disease as a homosexual one led to an attitude of "who cares," while a sense of political correctness on the part of the medical establishment kept the majority of physicians from being involved. The political and economic establishments turned their backs on the increasing number of AIDS patients, refusing to acknowledge that, in truth, the bell was tolling for them as well as for everyone else.

It was almost a decade to the day after the European gastroenterologists first noticed the fungal infections in the throats of patients that the world's infectious disease experts finally turned to virologists for help. In January of 1984 a physician at a conference discussing AIDS turned to the audience and asked, "Is there a retrovirologist in the house?"

20

If later in life you come to a fork in the road, take it.

YOGI BERRA

There were never more than two dozen retrovirologists in the world at any one time, and even those few were, at best, ignored by mainstream microbiology and, at worst, viewed with suspicion by other virologists. The study of retroviruses was indeed a very small research niche back in the 1980s. It was in every way a backwater of virology; the researchers devoted their energies and talents to the study of a tiny class of viruses that contained single strands of RNA and seemed in some way to be involved with malignancies. The RNA viruses were found to be the filterable agents in animal tumors. But no one understood how a virus containing only a strand of RNA could do *anything* to tissue, much less cause cancer. These viruses were viewed by most virologists as mere contaminants when they were found in malignant tissues; yet the few retrovirologists were convinced that these single-stranded RNA viruses were partially—if not totally—responsible for causing cancer.

It was an uphill fight at best. For nearly a hundred years, the accepted theory of tumor generation had centered solely on the exposure of human cells to known carcinogens. The idea that cancers occurred only after prolonged exposures to chemical carcinogens started in England with the study of skin cancers in chimney sweeps. It was observed that skin cancers occurred frequently in chimney sweeps but only after twenty to thirty years of constant exposure to the carbons and soot of furnaces and chimneys. The idea that exposure to carcinogens was a prerequisite to the production of any tumor was accepted as the rule rather than the exception. This theory was supported by the discovery that cigarette smoking leads to lung cancers and prolonged benzene exposure results in bladder tumors.

The discovery of the structure of DNA gave the carcinogenic exposure theory of cancer production the theoretical teeth it needed to take hold of both medicine's heart and mind. A cell's exposure to a known carcinogen was said to lead to alterations in the cell's DNA. The altered DNA led to damaged genes, which eventually led to loss of internal cellular control, and once control was lost, a malignant degeneration where the cell would take off on its own, liver cells becoming a hepatic tumor, epithelial cells in the lung producing a squamous cell carcinoma. The proponents of the carcinogenic view of cancer production used the long latency periods of exposure before malignancies developed to support their theory. Evidence that years of summer sunlight are needed to turn skin cells into basal cell carcinomas seemed to give credence and support to this prolonged-environmental-exposure view of cancer. No one thought to ask why such exposures required twenty to thirty years, or why everyone exposed to the same environmental carcinogens didn't develop the same cancers, or more to the point, why certain cancers seemed to run in certain families.

There was something understandable and intellectually satisfying, even if wrong, in the idea that normal, healthy cells exposed to daily doses of a foul poison would eventually have had enough and giving up, like some kind of drunken sailor, take off in the wrong direction. Besides, there was also something comforting in thinking that our cancers were not our fault but the result of polluting industries or some greedy landfill operator. A whole industry developed to support this view. Government agencies and private enterprises devised methods to check on the carcinogenic potential of almost every chemical, pesticide, and food additive. The proponents took the idea of exposure to substances as the cause of cancer into evaluations of normal foods, correlating degrees of national sugar consumption to the incidence of breast cancer, malignancies of the pancreas with the number of cups of coffee consumed per day, and stomach cancers to excessive intake of irritating or highly spiced foods.

It was a crazy time, but two retrovirologists, George J. Todara and Robert J. Huebner, taking comfort from the common sense notion that, "No one ever made a pig grow by weighing it," were sure that all these carcinogen exposure data were meaningless. Neither liked the explanations for the long latency periods proposed by the carcinogenicists, basically because the periods didn't make any biological sense. Why the need for decades of exposure? Why not a week or even a day? A delay of years, not to mention decades, did not support any biological theory of cellular alteration; but then again, retrovirologists understood that the cancer establishment did not like the idea that viruses might cause cancer and simply refused to accept any implication of the retroviruses.

But Huebner and Todara persisted. They added RNA viruses to what they had come to call "permissive" cell cultures, or cells that they knew could become malignant. They watched as the viral particles attached themselves to the cell walls and inserted their inner RNA core into the cell's cytoplasm; and then, as with all viral infections, this inner core containing the strands of nucleotides vanished. The disappearance was not unexpected; what happened to the cells next was. After the disappearance of the viral RNA, the cells continued to look, act, grow, and divide quite normally, until, after perhaps the twentieth cellular division, the cells suddenly started to take on strange shapes. Their nuclei swelled and, clearly out of control, began to divide wildly.

Todara and Huebner reasoned that the only possible explanation for the disappearance of the viral genes, followed eventually by the rapid degeneration of cellular control, was that the viral genes had gained some kind of basic chemical control—not enough to produce more viral particles, yet clearly enough to disrupt cellular function. The most logical explanation was that the viral genes had become incorporated into the permissive cell's own DNA and somehow, as had occurred in the primeval seas, been carried forward along with the cell's own DNA during each subsequent cellular division and that later, during one of the cell's many divisions, the viral nucleotides had become activated and had short-circuited the cell's own control mechanisms, turning the cell, like some kind of microscopic Frankenstein, into a biological monster.

Whatever finally kills a cancer patient—malnutrition, heart failure, infection, bleeding, or uremia—the characteristic common to all cancers is the loss of cellular control. It was clear from the early cancer studies that, like a real Frankenstein, malignant cells never revert to normal. Cancer cells are immortal; the passing on of the malignancy to each subsequent generation of new cells speaks of an irreversible change passed on to all future generations, and that could only mean a change in the cell's genetic code. In short, the only way to stop a malignant cell is to kill it.

But there were, of course, problems with Todara and Huebner's conclusion that infection with a retrovirus causes cancer. There was the usual concern about how single strands of RNA could reproduce themselves, much less be incorporated into the cell's own DNA, and there was the refusal of the cancer establishment, busy looking for environmental carcinogens, to admit that viruses might be a cause of cancer. The majority of virologists would say that poor George Todara and Robert Huebner were at best misguided and at worst wrong. It was pearls in wine and evaluating the intervention of the five inertia all over again. But the two retrovirologists had their observations and they had their data; and they were willing to compromise.

Todara and Huebner proposed that the long latency periods between carcinogenic exposures and the development of cancers could best be explained by the fact that the carcinogens activated the latent viral genes already incorporated into the cell's own DNA from a previous and perhaps unnoticed infection. They wrote in the *Proceedings of the National Academy of Sciences*:

> Several new lines of evidence have led us to propose that there exists a unique class of viruses [retroviruses] present in most, and perhaps in all, vertebrates that plays an important etiologic role in the development of tumors in these animals. The unique property of this virus group, we suggest, is that viral information can be transmitted from animal progeny to animal and from cell to progeny cell as a repressed viral genome. In this sense, these agents behave more like cellular genes than like infectious viruses; consequently, horizontal transmission (animal to animal and from cell to cell) is a natural mode of spread of cancer.

The two scientists had more than their own noncarcinogenic view of malignant degeneration. They had the predictable patterns of tumor development in certain families that clearly had nothing to do with exposure to carcinogens. Retinoblastoma is a malignant tumor of the eye that occurs in certain families. The cancer can affect both eyes, but children with both eyes involved all have close relatives with the same disease in one eye. The molecular biologists showed that in the single-eye disease, only one gene was abnormal; in bilateral tumors, two genes were damaged before the cells in the back of the eyes became overtly malignant. It seemed on close genetic analysis that the damaged genes were not human genes at all but the genes of a virus that humans had picked up during an earlier infection and that had become part of the human genome carried forward along with all the rest of the human genes to once again become associated in the cells of these cancer-prone families.

But the idea of *oncogenes*—genes made up of viral nucleotides hidden away in a cell's own DNA, replicated, and then carried forward into future cellular generations, ready to turn on at some future date and, like a hand grenade going off, so disrupt cellular function that the cell would eventually become malignant—was dismissed by a nervous medical community. Todara and Huebner might have been willing to give the cancer establishment their cigarettes, asbestos, dioxin, benzene, and ultraviolet rays, but only in association with their theory of oncogenes. They published again in the *Proceedings of The National Academy of Sciences*:

Viruses were first demonstrated to be oncogenic in chickens by Ellermann and Rous about sixty years ago and in mice by Gross in 1951. Since that time, but especially in the last few years, morphologically and functionally similar viruses have also been isolated from hamsters and cats, and have been seen, though infrequently, by electron microscopy in several other species including man. While the complete infectious form of the virus is rarely observed under natural conditions, in certain inbred mouse strains with high leukemia incidence, and some lines of chickens, overt virus is commonly observed and is demonstrable even prior to birth. In low or moderate leukemia-incidence mouse strains, overt [genetic] expression is generally absent early in life, but appears in certain tissues later at a time when there is also an increased incidence of tumors. Whether infectious virus and/or tumor becomes expressed is determined largely by host genetic factors, but expression can be influenced by environmental factors such as radiation and exposures to carcinogens.

Today's pediatric oncologists are well aware that the acute childhood leukemias result from acquired genetic lesions that activate cellular oncogenes or inactivate tumor-suppressor genes, leading to loss of growth control and that in these leukemias, exchanges of genetic information between chromosomes are frequently responsible for converting cellular genes to oncogenes or activated viral genes by repositioning them at new chromosomal sites.

But today's scientists have taken the idea of viral genes as parts of human DNA a step further, or in a way, a step backward. There are groups of researchers who now consider that viral infections may have contributed to cellular evolution. These molecular geneticists consider that throughout evolution it was the constant infusion of new viral genes into an organism's genetic code that provided cells with a constant supply of new and different genes, giving these organisms new possibilities to cope with a changing environment and provide the adaptations necessary in a competitive world. It is possible that the sudden ability of a cell to transform one protein into another or to bind calcium carbonate did not come about by a mutation in the cell's own genetic code but from an infection with a virus whose own nucleotide base pair sequences, inserted into the genes of the infected cell, changed that cell's blueprint, the new hybrid genetic code allowing for a new, more dynamic cell better able to prosper and survive.

Genes, viruses, cancer, cellular control, immunology, evolution, life, and death: By the middle 1980s, they were coming together, and where they met was at the lymphocyte.

21

Increase your knowledge, or you will decrease it.

THE MISHNA

The discovery of B lymphocytes gave immunologists enormous problems. They were much like the chemists of Pasteur's time trying to explain Mitscherlich planes before there was any understanding of optical isomers. Immunologists knew that the B lymphocytes produced antibodies, but they couldn't explain how these cells were able to form the hundreds, if not thousands, of specific antibodies necessary over a lifetime to defend against real as well as potential attackers.

In short, the immunologists could not explain what was called "the enigma of antibody diversity." Some researchers believed there was an all-purpose antibody, a "one size fits all" scenario. Others proposed that somehow the large number of circulating lymphocytes each producing an individual antibody guaranteed that sooner or later the right antibody would be produced. Both scenarios had their obvious problems. The first was simply foolish; the second demanded that lymphocytes contain specific antibody-producing genes that somehow anticipated any and all future microbial attacks. It was the primeval seas, chaos, complexity, and the demands of survival coupled to mathematical probabilities all over again.

There simply could never be enough individual genes to make all the necessary antibodies to defend against every possible new microscopic invader that an individual might encounter throughout a lifetime, and that concern was without taking into account the fact that bacteria and viruses are themselves undergoing their own mutations.

In the 1970s, two Japanese biologists, studying antibody production in lymphocytes that had undergone a malignant transformation, proved that in leukemias the malignant cells construct antibodies from different nucleotide segments that are shifted around within the single antibody coding gene. It was clear from these studies that malignant lymphocytes have the ability to shift parts, even whole genes, inside their nucleus and use the different combinations and sequences to produce any number of different antibodies.

Researchers used the Japanese techniques to study normal antibody production and found that what was true of cancerous lymphocytes was also true of normal B lymphocytes. The answer to antibody diversity lies in the genes and the ability at the subcellular level of cells to shift around the segments of their own genes. The complexity of evolution does indeed verge on chaos; and nowhere is this more clearly seen than in the enormous investment of life in antibody protection and the fact that the investment began at the very beginning of cellular evolution. Sponges, the earliest and simplest of multicellular creatures, produce proteins that will attack tissue grafts from other sponges, while earthworms, in addition to the scavenging phagocytes patrolling their tissues, produce very primitive molecules called "lectins" that act like antibodies and bind to different molecules. Different types of lectins isolated from sea urchins and flying insects bind to surface sugars different from the sugars making up their own cells' surfaces. Hemolin, a protein isolated from the tissue fluids of moths, has gone one step further and will bind to nonsugar structures in the cell walls of bacteria. But however early the production of antibodylike proteins, today's modern antibodies are constructed of two distinct genetically coded amino acid chains—a short and a long chain. Each B lymphocyte has at least twenty genes available in its nucleus to produce the two parts of an antibody molecule. A circulating lymphocyte carrying the information of an attacking bacterium back to the nearest lymph node is much like a honeybee returning to its hive to give the other bees the information on location, distance, and azi-muth to the nearest flower bed. The returning lymphocyte presents the information about the stranger's surface to the other cells in the lymph nodes. Those "hive-bound" B cells quickly release their own nuclear enzymes, which break the links in the antibody coding regions on their chromosomes, allowing the freed gene segments to randomly rearrange themselves in different configurations. These rearranged segments, when reconnected, establish a new, unique antibody coding unit that precisely fits the copy of the surface marker brought back by the circulating lymphocytes.

The numbers are on the side of survival. In a population of billions of B cells, millions of new cells being added each day to replace the millions that die or wear out, the mathematical possibilities of quickly producing an antibody that will fit the new surface become better than one to one. At any time, during any one moment, the body's lymphocytes have the potential by rearranging their twenty genes to produce more than 10^{14} different antibodies, more antibodies than the number of galaxies in the universe. Add to all this the random rearrangements and the occurrence of a mutation in any one of the twenty gene segments, and the number of different antibodies available at any one time to bind to a foreign surface overwhelms the possibility of any foreign surface escaping detection or of eluding antibody binding and attack by the body's immune system. Molecular biologists have shown that a change or shift of only one amino acid in an antibody can increase the binding ability of an antibody to a specific foreign surface by a factor of over 1,000. The odds for survival lie with the defender. But this obsession with surfaces, the ability of one cell to make a protein that specifically binds to a receptor site on another, has proven to be even more fundamental to life than defense.

Recently researchers discovered a gene on chromosome 7 coding for the construction of a surface receptor on the cell walls of all the cells lining the small intestine that specifically binds molecules of vitamin D. The binding of vitamin D to these receptor sites is an absolute requirement for the body to absorb dietary calcium. The locking of a molecule of vitamin D into the receptor site on the cells making up the surface of our intestines acts as a switch that turns on enzymes within the tissues of the intestine to increase the absorption of calcium from milk and milk products.

The disease of osteoporosis, the brittle bone condition mostly affecting older women, is in reality a genetic disease. As a woman ages, the gene governing the production of the vitamin D receptor sites forms a defective receptor that keeps molecules of vitamin D from properly fitting into cell membranes, leading to a decrease in absorption of dietary calcium and the development of osteoporosis. There have been other confusing diseases involving bones and calcium. One called hypocalcemic hypercalciuria is a familial condition, transmitted from parent to child, that presents in the teenage years with low serum calcium, seizures, and spasms. In order to treat the low calcium levels, physicians are forced to use large doses of vitamin D, which leads to kidney stones and renal failure. Analysis of these patients' DNA has showed a mutation located on chromosome 3 that codes for a new cell surface protein of 1,078 amino acids in length, specifically, a calcium-sensing receptor that is necessary for the body to maintain normal levels of serum calcium.

But the new ability to study the genetic code itself has implications for medicine that go quite beyond a better understanding of disease or the mere sorting out of more effective therapies. This revolution, like sanitation systems and the discovery of anesthesia and immunizations, has profound implications for all of us. Each day, 15,000 Americans turn fifty; by the year 2010, 40 to 65 million Americans will be between the ages of fifty and seventy-five. Each day a larger and larger group of men will awake with decreased sexual desire, decreased bone density, a decreasing lean body mass, and increasing mental confusion. The question, as it has always been in medicine, is why; and the answer, not unexpectedly, has been found to lie in our cells.

The molecular biologists are now able to accurately measure testosterone levels and find that as men age, circulating levels of this hormone begin to decrease. But testosterone is a "signal" protein, part of the latch and key mechanism of cellular communication . . . lose the key and you lose the message. In one of the early studies on aging, synthetic testosterone was given to men known to have decreased levels of this hormone and the researchers found that in a significant number libido increased, lean body mass improved, and bones hardened. Receptor sites for molecules of testosterone have been found in the cell walls of the prostate gland as well as the cells of other tissues, including muscle, bone, and the cells of the central nervous system. In short, the new genetic revolution will no longer deal solely with external threats or internal pathology but with how we feel and how we think.

It was this lock-and-key means of communication arising in the primeval seas that became the conversation of choice between cells and their tissues and not only for protection but for general awareness as well as command and control.

Pain itself is an example of just how effective and yet how simple this "bootstrapping" has become. Whatever else pain may be, it begins with the activation of our nervous system: Cut your finger and you pull your hand back; touch a burning object and you jump back. Early in evolution, nature hit on a fail-proof method of survival. What is the one molecule present in every living cell? Indeed, what is the one function necessary to maintain life? It is the ability to store and use energy. Forget to put gas in your car and you can't go anywhere; lose the electricity to your neighborhood and the house shuts down. You may not even be able to get in or out of your garage. Cellular integrity and tissue function need energy. Early in evolution a molecule, *adenosine triphosphate* (ATP), a very simple molecule, took on the ability to store energy in its triphosphate bonds, releasing the energy on demand. It is such an ancient molecule that it exists in every living cell. Some cells contain chlorophyll; some, muscle proteins; some make insulin; but every cell contains ATP. Pain is always related to tissue damage, so it was inevitable that as nerves were integrated into evolving organisms and they developed the ability to respond to tissue damage, the fail-safe system of response would be the release of molecules of ATP. The syllogism is quite clear: ATP exists only in cells; if ATP is found outside of a cell, specifically in the fluids surrounding a nerve ending, the cells in the vicinity of the nerve must have been ripped or torn.

In fact, there are receptor sites at the ends of nerves that are specific for binding the molecules of ATP. Released ATP fits into the ATP receptors at the end of nerves. If ATP is injected into skin, people feel the same pain as if they had been cut or burned. There are neurologists who realize that the treatment of pain no longer has to rely solely on the use of the morphines but find ways to block the ATP receptor sites at the nerve endings so that released molecules of ATP no longer fit. Indeed, the real treatment of pain will lie in the sequencing of the gene that constructs the ATP nerve end receptor and then developing the ability to interfere with that blueprint so that the receptors are never made or are constructed in such a way that ATP never fits into them and the whole sequence of pain production never begins.

But what nature gives, nature also takes away. This molecular lock-and-key effect is too powerful and pervasive a tool to be given up if and when there is the occasional mistake, or misreading of the key. While medical students are still taught the six categories of disease, there remains a seventh classification that reaches into all six and yet remains distinct. The conditions where the body attacks itself—rheumatoid arthritis, myasthenia gravis, lupus erythematosus, multiple sclerosis, dermatomyositis, Hashimoto's thyroiditis are just a few of these autoimmune diseases.

When the conversations between the body's immune system and its own different surfaces become garbled, the cells of the immune system misread surface proteins on perfectly normal cells as abnormal or "nonself." Diabetes has had a rather checkered history. Once thought to be congenital, then infectious and metabolic, it is now considered to be an autoimmune disease. The disease begins with the destruction of the patient's islet cells, cells embedded in the pancreas that produce insulin. When these cells are damaged, circulating insulin levels decrease and blood glucose levels rise as muscles are inhibited from absorbing sugar. The patient becomes weak and dehydrated. Biopsies of islet cells, like the biopsies of the skin from Medawar mice, show destruction of the islet cells by the body's immune system.

But why should a patient's immune system misread the surface markers of its own islet cells? Recently researchers have discovered an association between drinking cow's milk in childhood and the later development of diabetes. What these scientists found was that some milk proteins are quite similar to the proteins making up the cell walls of islet cells. Immunologists have mixed the lymphocytes of diabetics with milk proteins and these lymphocytes recognize the proteins as foreign. The very fact that cow's milk proteins are similar to the proteins on the surface of islet cells, and that lymphocytes recognize the similarities, is just another indication that nature discards nothing, and uses all that it has from one phase-shift to another.

Once the body misreads the message, its macrophages, neutrophils, and lymphocytes attack with the same single-minded ferocity that they would use attacking an invading bacterium, virus, or transplanted tissue. But nowhere is the havoc of the body turning against itself more clearly or dramatically demonstrated than in the desperate history of a six-year-old boy admitted recently to Massachusetts General Hospital after three days of fatigue, nausea, and vomiting, followed by tingling in his legs that quickly advanced to weakness and the inability to walk and then death. It is a cautionary tale.

The child had spent the week before his admission to the hospital at a summer camp where he rode horses. The parents were unaware of any tick bites and reported that their son had eaten no shellfish or other seafood prior to admission.

The child's white blood cell count on admission to the infectious disease ward was markedly elevated. A spinal tap was done, revealing spinal fluid that was cloudy and containing 1,200 white cells per ml, 90 percent of which were neutrophils and 10 percent lymphocytes. A diagnosis of meningitis was made and antibiotics were administered intravenously. But despite the antibiotics, the child continued to do poorly. A CT scan of the child's head revealed findings consistent with swelling of the right hemisphere of the brain. On the second day of hospitalization the child's heart began to fail and he was placed on mechanical cardiac and respiratory support. Surprisingly, the spinal fluid cultures were negative. No other bacteria were found. The diagnosis of bacterial meningitis was clearly in doubt. On the fourth hospital day, the child became comatose. There was no response to pain and all deep tendon reflexes were absent. A radionuclide brain scan revealed no evidence of blood flow to the brain, no obvious cortical or brain perfusion. Later that day the child was pronounced dead.

The child had clearly died a central nervous system death, beginning with a paralysis of his legs that progressed within four days to virtually the complete destruction of the child's brain. The central question that faced the physicians taking care of this child and that later became the pivotal issue in understanding what had caused the child's death was whether there had been a direct virial infection of the child's central nervous system or some kind of autoimmune reaction.

Eastern equine encephalitis was a possibility. Certain enteroviruses can infect both the heart and the brain; but the usual signs of a viral encephalitis—abrupt onset of high fever, neck rigidity, headaches, disorientation, and altered level of consciousness—were simply not present; and the child's CT scan results did not match the focal lesions caused by the virus. And of course the presence of so many neutrophils in the child's spinal fluid was not consistent with the immune response to a virus, which always involves large numbers of lymphocytes. There was also the fact that the child's neurological problems began in his legs and appeared to work up into the brain. Lyme disease can affect the central nervous system and was considered, but the rapidly fatal course in what had been a healthy child was considered unusual for Lyme disease.

The three facts that had to be explained were the child's rapidly fatal course, inability to grow or find any signs of an infectious agent, and the enormous number of neutrophils in the child's spinal fluid. An Internet search of the medical literature showed that between 1940 and 1960 six patients had been reported who had died of "an acute cerebral condition." All were associated with a rapidly fatal course and the presence of large numbers of neutrophils in their spinal fluids. All these patients were noted to have had a preceding mild viral illness followed almost immediately by paralysis and death. No viruses were found in the brains of these patients, nor was a virus found at autopsy in the brain of the child; all that was found was the destruction of nerve cells and the presence of the huge numbers of neutrophils.

It has recently become clear that relatively benign viruses may, during the course of a flulike illness, somehow damage nervous tissue, altering surface proteins or releasing small amounts of brain cell proteins into the spinal fluid or circulation. In most cases, nothing comes of this; the patient has a few days of coughing, a headache, muscle tenderness and the illness passes and the patient recovers. But in some patients, perhaps those few with a hyperactive immune system or a genetically altered lock-and-key mechanism, the damaged nervous system surface markers or released intracellular proteins sequestered away inside the brain cells are suddenly recognized as "foreign" and the full weight of the immune system is set in motion to attack and destroy what in reality are completely normal cells. In this terrible example of "friendly fire," killer T cells migrate into the nervous tissue, releasing their cytokines that not only recruit other T cells but huge numbers of circulating neutrophils, which flood into the area, triggering massive tissue destruction.

Experimental neurologists took these observations a step further and began a number of studies much like Koch's tuberculin injection studies a hundred years earlier, involving the injection of parts of nerve cells into rats. The researchers found that such injections did cause immune destruction of the rat's central nervous system. In the early 1980s it was found, both in humans and experimental animals, that a very small number of activated T lymphocytes can recognize markers on damaged brain cells as "foreign," inducing and then amplifying an inflammatory response in the central nervous system that can destroy normal tissue.

The edge of medical research is now out at the borders of gene function, surface markers, mediators, cytokines, lymphocyte interaction, antigen processing, and receptor sites. These interconnections became more sinister when virologists discovered that viruses use their own outer protein coats as attachment sites for specific cell surface markers. It appears that early in evolution, viruses took advantage of developing cellular life by adapting their outer surfaces to fit the outer surfaces of evolving cells, just as surely as the smaller dinosaurs of the early Jurassic age turned their forelimbs into wings to take advantage of the empty skies.

The idea of specific receptor sites became even more ominous when it was discovered that the first immune abnormality in patients with AIDS is a decrease in the number of their circulating lymphocytes, and not just any group of lymphocytes, but a specific subset of T lymphocytes, those with the CD4 receptors on their surfaces.

22

You cannot have justice without order.

FEDERALIST PAPERS

There have always been turf wars in medicine. The attacks on Paracelsus, Semmelweis, Harvey, Pasteur, Jenner, and Marshall had more to do with the medical establishment refusing to jeopardize their own position than any reasoned challenge to new ideas. Today, in the world of facial reconstruction, the plastic surgeons fight it out for patients with ear, nose, and throat specialists, while family practice doctors employed by managed health care companies belittle the need for subspecialists, while the subspecialists complain that the generalists "are so well rounded that they point in no direction at all."

Cancer, too, has had its turf wars. President Nixon's $100 million war on cancer was fought over by the surgeons with their cut-and-slash techniques as well as by the oncologists pushing their poison-and-burn methods. But today, drawn together by the retrovirologists, the molecular biologists, and the geneticists, a consensus concerning cancer—and, in fact, all malignancies—is beginning to form. No one likes it. The surgeons are uncomfortable because it takes the scalpel out of their hands;

the oncologists dislike it because it points the way toward the absolute futility of all their injection and medication protocols; and the health-care insurance companies and politicians worry that it will all be terribly expensive.

It is the view that the malignant transformation of a cell is not a single event but a progression of evolutionary cells that eventually yields a variant with new cellular properties of movement and invasiveness as well as unrestrained and unregulated growth. There is no doubt that the pressure of evolution still exists within any individual cell as it does within any complete organism. Indeed, it is this pressure to change that leads to both disaster and survival. In complex organisms, all cells are under continuous pressure to mutate, to grow to better themselves in order to give the edge to their own, but this runs the risk of going too far, of causing disruptive dangerous alterations.

There has to be a kind of balance here. Organisms maintain the edge, while preventing overt malignant transformations and the production of abnormal or damaging proteins, by putting subcellular systems in place to ensure accurate DNA replication, including the ability to repair any abnormally spliced DNA, and if that fails, the ability in a process of cellular suicide to kill off any severely mutated cell. That the systems work so well is astonishing, that mistakes occur, a virtual inevitability. There are now at least 500 medical and surgical conditions, from cystic fibrosis to the various forms of hemophilia, that are known to be caused by alterations to the genetic code.

It is clear today that mutations, gene deletions, viral insertions, chromosomal translocations, and duplications of any one of 200 different genes contribute to tumor formation. Somewhere during the evolution of multicellular organisms, and even before such development, cellular mechanisms had to be constructed to get rid of the "bad apples." It wouldn't serve the evolving amphibians to have each of their pancreatic islet cells go its own way and stop making insulin.

In the search of such a control system, the molecular biologists have found a gene, labeled P53, existing in all living things, including yeasts, that is "the guardian of the genome." It is a gene that encodes for the production of a nuclear protein that binds to and regulates the cellular enzymes that repair damaged DNA. There are now hundreds of articles in obscure and little-read journals such as *Trends in Genetics, British Journal of Cancer, American Journal of Human Genetics, Oncogene, Cell,* and the *Proceedings of the National Academy of Sciences* proving not only that abnormalities and deletions in this P53 gene occur in over 80 percent of all human colon cancers and 40 percent of breast tumors and that those malignancies that do have abnormal or nonfunctioning P53 genes are the most aggressive and unstable cancers and the most resistant to therapy.

The P53 gene lies on chromosome 17 along with other "policing genes" that physically stabilize chromosomes while ordering normal cellular division and intertissue growth.

The P53 gene is absolutely necessary for normal cell growth and differentiation. Animals with a defective P53 gene are normal at birth but develop tumors quite early from mutations that occur in their rapidly dividing cells, some of which, because of rapid proliferation, develop breaks in their DNA. Exposure to high-energy radiation, sunlight, or chemical carcinogens, is known to damage DNA. A defect in the cell's P53 gene clearly short-circuits the cell's damage control capabilities and ability to repair its DNA. It appears that damaged DNA stimulates the production of the P53 gene to produce a nuclear protein that stops any further DNA production, leading to growth arrest in the cell with the damaged chromosome, literally shutting down the whole cell, allowing the abnormal sections of DNA to be serviced and, if necessary, replaced. If the DNA cannot be repaired, the P53 gene, by continuing to produce its nuclear protein, keeps the damaged cell in a state of suspended animation until it dies or is destroyed by the immune system. What the molecular biologists have proven beyond any doubt is that an absence of the P53 gene, or a mutation in its base pairs that yields the production of an abnormal nuclear protein, is precisely the same as having a community with no police available to stop or arrest the crazed or the criminal. In fact, most malignant cells do contain a defective version of the P53 protein. Chemotherapies and radiations designed to kill cancer cells by damaging their DNA have a great deal more trouble destroying malignant cells deficient in the P53 gene product, presumably because these cells have lost, whatever the damage, the main control switch to shut down. With the P53 gene gone, malignant cells simply won't die, despite being poisoned, because even the mechanisms that lead to cell death are no longer present. A cell with an absent or damaged P53 gene is truly an immortal cell that will go on living and dividing, squeezing out the tissues and organs that patients need to live until eventually the malignancy and the patient both die.

Disease and death: It is all down now where it has always been—at the subcellular level where DNA reproduces itself and bridges the gap between chemistry and life.

23

*I don't know what the enemy thinks of our troops,
but they sure scare the hell out of me.*

THE DUKE OF WELLINGTON

There is little doubt today that AIDS began in Africa. By December of 1983 the disease had spread throughout most of the central area of the continent. French and Belgian physicians searching through hospital records and death certificates not only proved the origin of the disease in the remote villages along Lake Victoria but documented its spread through the equatorial nations. The data showed that the disease killed equal numbers of men and women and that the typical female patient was a young married woman. The typical male victims were somewhat older men who had had numerous sexual partners.

The African epidemic spread along the newly constructed highways and transportation systems linking the rural areas to the developing towns and cities. Some epidemiologists have suggested that the cause of the rapid spread of the disease was the new mobility of the African people.

There has been some controversy about both the exact origin and the method of spreading AIDS, but as with all sexually trans-

THE LIGHT IN THE SKULL · 171

mitted diseases it allowed the guardians of morality and social standards to begin to weave their own self-serving webs of confusion and indifference. If AIDS were cholera there would be no real debate, no obfuscating of the real issues or the real facts; people would look at the data and simply do what had to be done.

The retrovirologist in America who was finally persuaded to help pursue the viral cause of AIDS was Robert Gallo, of the National Institutes of Health. In France it was Luc Montagnier, of the Pasteur Institute. Gallo, a meticulous researcher whose own sister had died of lymphatic leukemia, had developed a lifelong interest in cancers of the lymphatic system, devoting most of his professional life to the study of virus-induced malignancies. Gallo had isolated a growth factor that, when added to cultures of lymphocytes, kept those cells alive and healthy for both experimental manipulation and viral isolation. Montagnier, too, was interested in the development of leukemias in particular and malignancies in general.

Gallo had helped the Japanese in the study of their own epidemics of leukemia. The Japanese physicians wondered if these leukemia patients were infected with a virus and asked Gallo to help them study their patients. After a great deal of effort, Gallo was able to grow a single-strand RNA virus from the leukemic cells of these patients. In a series of brilliant experiments he proved that the virus not only attached specifically to the T-cell subset of lymphocytes in these patients but that the virus was indeed the cause of their leukemias.

Gallo named the virus HTLV, for human T-cell leukemia virus. He published his findings in an article entitled "Human T-Cell Leukemia-Lymphoma Virus (HTLV) Is in T- but not B-Lymphocytes from a Patient with Cutaneous T-Cell Lymphoma." The discovery of a virus that caused leukemia should have been an achievement worthy of a Nobel Prize, but the idea of a virus causing tumors was considered so outrageous that the article was attacked. The reviewers complained that Gallo had not proved that the virus was anything more than a contaminant in the cell's cytoplasm, challenging his whole contention that this RNA virus was the cause of this specific leukemia, much less of any human malignancy. An RNA virus simply had no place in the accepted scheme of evolution or of biology. How did it replicate itself, how did it survive, and how did it incorporate its RNA into the lymphocyte's DNA? Gallo's work was dismissed by everyone but the Japanese who, thanking Gallo, began to look for a leukemia vaccine.

Gallo ignored the attacks and continued his pursuit of the virus. He studied the lymphocytes and blood serums of the families of the Japanese patients with T-cell leukemias and made a disquieting discovery. He found antibodies to his newly isolated virus in the plasma from some of the wives of the leukemia patients. Since the antibodies he found were specific for the HTLV virus, Gallo had no choice but to conclude that these women, while still clinically healthy, had been infected and might still be harboring the virus somewhere in their bodies. Gallo understood that in order for the women, indeed any person, to develop a specific antibody to HTLV, the virus had to have entered their circulation and come into contact with their own lymphocytes. Gallo wrote another article dealing with the discovery of these antibodies, ending with what would prove to be a prophetic note, "The results indicate that [HTLV] was not transmitted through the germ line, but rather acquired by infection." It was not that Dr. Gallo had caught up with the real world, but that the real world was catching up with Dr. Gallo.

While Gallo was making his discoveries concerning the viral involvement in human T-cell leukemias, there was an acrimonious meeting of the administrators of the California Blood Bank Association. At the meeting, representatives of homosexual groups challenged a proposal by a number of infectious disease experts who recommended that blood donors be checked for sexual preference. The homosexuals demanded that no direct or indirect questions about a potential blood donor's sexuality be part of any donor questionnaire. The challenge simply showed the craziness occurring on both sides of the AIDS issue. What should first and foremost have been a medical issue had become a cultural and a political one. It was to become an issue on which only the retrovirologists would turn out to be right.

Two other virologists, James Timmons and David Baltimore, were to find the one piece of evidence that would silence Gallo's critics and become the single most important clue in solving the riddle that was AIDS. They were studying the structure of the single-stranded RNA viruses and made an astonishing discovery that would give this species of viruses a name all their own: the *retroviruses*. Timmons and Baltimore found that the inner core of these viruses contained not only the expected single nucleotide strand of RNA but also a much tinier strand of amino acids in the inner core, physically packaged right next to the RNA.

It was so simple and so clever that it was elegant. This tiny polypeptide made up of a strand of only twenty-two amino acids, on its own, literally reverses the whole process of evolution. Timmons and Baltimore discovered that this tiny enzyme works backwards and actually forms a normal double helical strand of DNA from the virus's single strand of RNA. At one time this enzyme evolving along with replicating polymers and membranes must have become the new player in town, a player that developed the ability to reverse all the evolution that had gone on before and would come after. Timmons and Baltimore called this small polypeptide "reverse transcriptase." A particle of reverse transcriptase will allow a single strand of RNA to form a complementary strand of DNA, which then goes on to form the usual double helix carrying in the newly constructed DNA the code from the single strand of RNA. In the growing complexity of evolution, this strange group of RNA viruses had found their own prescription for survival: work backwards.

During an infection with a retrovirus, the virus not only injects its genetic code into the cell's interior but also its segment of reverse transcriptase. The RNA of a retrovirus contains four genes: a gene that codes for the production of the virus's outer coat; a second for the production of its inner membrane; a third that codes for the manufacture of particles of reverse transcriptase; and a fourth gene, called the "assembly gene," which produces an enzyme that assembles all four parts, including a replica of the original RNA, into a complete virus.

The particles of reverse transcriptase are so important to the survival of RNA viruses that during the final assembly process a particle of reverse transcriptase is always incorporated first into the viral core, even before the strand of RNA. The packaging of this preformed enzyme within each viral particle guarantees that once the virus infects a new cell its code will be quickly translated and inserted into the cell's own DNA, to be carried forward into all future generations of the infected cell. In some cells the incorporation of a retroviral genome into a cell's DNA does not lead first to more viruses but rather to these cells losing control and becoming overtly malignant.

The discovery of reverse transcriptase was the smoking gun that proved that RNA viruses, once inside a cell, could incorporate their genetic code into the cell's own genetic material.

In 1985 both Gallo, at the National Institutes of Health, and Luc Montagnier, in Paris, were totally committed to finding the answer to AIDS. But even with their considerable skills things did not go well. They knew all about retroviruses but they couldn't find any in the bodies or in any specific cells of the AIDS patients.

Gallo began his experiments by trying to grow a virus from the circulating lymphocytes removed from AIDS patients. Since the earliest observable change in an AIDS patient's immune system was a decrease in the number of circulating lymphocytes, he had assumed that the lymphocytes would be the best place to look for the virus. He was singularly unsuccessful. Gallo simply could not get a retrovirus to grow in his cell cultures. In fact, all the cells in his tissue cultures died. The French at the Pasteur Institute were coming to the same dead end, literally; not only could they not grow a virus but, like Gallo, their lymphocyte tissue cultures all died too. Gallo could not explain the deaths of his cultures, but he began to doubt that a retrovirus was the cause of AIDS. After all, every retrovirus that had ever been discovered had been involved with the production of tumors and leukemias. Retroviruses did not cause cells to die; in fact, they did the opposite—they caused cells to divide and grow at abnormal rates. Still, Gallo continued to try to culture a virus from the lymphocytes of AIDS patients, though with less and less enthusiasm.

The French researchers took another path. Montagnier and his colleagues wondered if the decrease in circulating lymphocytes might not in reality be a secondary event. The earliest clinical observation in a patient with AIDS, other than a typical though short-lived flulike episode of achiness and a sore throat, was an early, persistent enlargement of the patient's lymph nodes. Perhaps, the French theorized, this generalized lymphadenopathy was in reality the primary biological event and the decrease in circulating lymphocytes a secondary consequence of infected lymph nodes, rather than the cause. The French decided to culture the lymph nodes of their AIDS patients instead of what remained of their circulating lymphocytes.

Montagnier asked the Institute physicians to remove a lymph node from an AIDS patient and send the tissue down to the retrovirology laboratory, where he placed sections of the node in a culture dish of healthy lymphocytes. The cells in the culture survived a few days and then, as had happened before, started to die.

Gallo's experiments in the United States had, however, shown one thing. Even though he was unable to grow a virus, Gallo did find small amounts of reverse transcriptase in the dying tissue culture cells. The presence of reverse transcriptase, the signature of a retrovirus, was confusing. But the assay technique was so sensitive that the discovery of such a small amount of the enzyme in a cell culture could easily be only a contaminant or a false positive. Gallo did, however, tell the French about finding the small amounts of reverse transcriptase.

Montagnier was about to cancel his own testing when, in one of those totally unexplainable moments of science, Montagnier's colleague, Françoise Barre-Sinoussi, a physician who had once herself studied with Gallo, did something quite remarkable. She did not dismiss the minute amounts of reverse transcriptase that Gallo had reported as meaningless data. She trusted in science and assumed that where there was reverse transcriptase, a retrovirus had to be present. As the cell cultures began to die, she added fresh, healthy lymphocytes to the culture plates, and as these cells began to die, she added more lymphocytes and began checking the dishes for the presence of reverse transcriptase. There were, as Gallo had said, small amounts of the enzyme present in the cultures. But after a week, Barre-Sinoussi found increasing amounts of the enzyme. As she added more and more lymphocytes, the amounts of reverse transcriptase continued to in-crease—doubling, tripling, and then quadrupling. It became clear to her that she had a retrovirus growing in her cultures. But if it was a retrovirus, it was one that no one had ever seen before. It was a virus that killed the cells it infected and, in killing the cell, killed itself. It seemed as if a crazed genetic fox had somehow entered the heart of the chicken coop.

24

*A change in only one of the thousands of bases
in a gene is enough to disrupt or completely
eliminate the gene product from the cell.*

GENETIC CONFERENCE

The French discovery of increasing amounts of reverse transcriptase in their dying cell cultures forced the virologists to conclude, however reluctantly, that they had discovered a new retrovirus, a retrovirus so astonishingly lethal that it killed lymphocytes virtually as soon as the cells were infected. The discovery of the reverse transcriptase caused both Gallo and Montagnier to redouble their efforts to grow the virus. Gallo thought he might have a way to do it. It was a long shot, but theoretically it might work, and it did.

Like Mendel pruning his fields of yellow and green peas, Gallo struggled on a fantastically smaller scale to cultivate a lymphocyte cell line that would survive the new virus. He assumed that already cancerous cells, cells that he knew were notoriously difficult to kill, might better survive the onslaught of a new virus and began to assay several neoplastic human cell lines for susceptibility to infection. When the cell proliferation declined, fresh cells derived from human lymphoid leukemia patients were added. After a number of twenty-hour-a-day weeks he was successful. As Gallo wrote in a report published in the journal *Cell:*

> The viability of different cells ranged from 65 to 85 percent and the doubling time of the cell population was approximately thirty to forty hours. Thus, our data showed that this permanently growing [leukemic] T-cell population can [survive] and continually produce virus.

There has been a meaningless argument filled with academic acrimony and sustained by petty confrontations about who first isolated the AIDS virus. While the issue was finally settled in favor of the French, neither the Americans nor the French could have found this confusing and deadly virus, much less grown it, without a decade of work and the help and discoveries of hundreds of other scientists, from the embryologists to the molecular geneticists. The real issues, the only issues, were the ability to finally grow the virus and, by applying Koch's postulates, to prove that indeed a retrovirus was the cause of the disease, as well as to have enough virus available to be able to examine its structure, how it works, in hope of devising a test to determine its presence and possible treatments and a vaccine.

That was the hope, but at first this new virus proved too nimble, too clever for anything except a blood test. It appeared that with AIDS, Dr. Seale's admonition that the worst of all possible worlds for a viral epidemic would be a cross-species transfer of a lethal virus with a prolonged incubation period has become a reality. The antibody test that was devised in Gallo's laboratory allowed blood banks to screen the nation's blood supply, but for individuals in 1986, or today, a positive test result would ultimately be a death sentence.

The ability to finally grow the AIDS virus gave the world an unlimited supply of virus to examine and study. A great deal has been learned. The AIDS virus is roughly spherical in shape and approximately one ten-thousandth of a millimeter across. Its outer coat contains numerous proteins, one protein consisting of four chains of amino acids, GP120, the *GP* standing for *glycoprotein* and the number referring to the mass of the protein measured in thousands of daltons. The virus uses its GP120 protein to attach itself to CD4 receptor sites on cell walls. Beneath the viral outer core there is an inner core constructed of two additional proteins, P17 and P24, containing two single strands of RNA each approximately 9,200 nucleotide bases long and, as expected, a piece of the enzyme reverse transcriptase. Also present in the core is another peptide enzyme, integrase, found to have the ability to splice a DNA copy of the viral RNA into the host cell's genetic material. It is all terribly simple and quite deadly.

Virologists have even been able to describe precisely how the virus replicates and how its enzymes work. The clearest explanation was written in *The Lancet*:

> The first thing that happens to the two strands of RNA in a newly infected cell is that their encoded message is converted into DNA by multiple reverse transcriptase molecules attached to the viral RNA. The process is the opposite of normal transcription, which makes RNA from DNA. [The enzyme] reverse transcriptase moves along the [strand of] RNA, producing an equivalent chain of DNA by sticking together the nucleotide building blocks. When the first DNA strand is complete, the reverse transcriptase starts constructing a second DNA strand, using the first one as a template.
>
> The reverse transcriptase that the AIDS virus uses is not very accurate: on average it introduces an error, or mutation, approximately every 2,000 incorporated nucleotides. . . . This intrinsic infidelity underlies the virus' remarkable ability to become resistant to various drugs [and any potential vaccines] because new variants of viral proteins are constantly generated during the course of an infection. . . . The two DNA strands produced by the reverse transcriptase are integrated by the integrase present near the reverse transcriptase. . . . Once one of the two strands of DNA have been incorporated into the host cell's chromosomes, the strands are

known as a "provirus" and the infection of the cell is permanent. . . . [The provirus] makes copies of messenger RNAs . . . and
viral replication begins and with the replication, cell death.

But all this information has done little to stop the worldwide
transmission of the virus or develop any effective cheap and easily accessible treatments. The truth is that cellular evolution has
never learned to handle retroviruses very well.

There is no doubt now that the AIDS virus belongs to a
strange genus of RNA viruses called *Lentivirus*. As a group, lenti-
viruses are known to have long incubation periods and, once activated, they do indeed kill the cells they have infected. The
AIDS virus also shows some characteristics similar to the simian
lymphotropic virus, a virus known for decades to cause a rather
benign disease in the green monkey of central Africa.

The assertion has been made that AIDS has always been a
human disease in Africa, resulting from the occasional inadvertent bite of a green monkey, but with the isolation of the earlier
African villager and no blood transfusion system or illicit drug
culture to spread the virus, as well as the possibility that the infected person might perhaps be a child, a sexually inactive adult,
or a monogamous husband, the disease may well have remained
a localized, individual affair from beginning to end. The explanation is not so farfetched, particularly when one begins to dissect
the issues of infections and host responses.

There is good reason to assume that when the AIDS virus
first attacked the green monkeys or, more accurately, their ancestors, the disease was as devastating as its attacks on humans
are today. It is quite likely that the majority of the original monkeys were killed and that the monkeys that exist today are the
direct descendants of those few survivors. The mildness of the
present-day primate disease is an example of a general immune
resistance passed on to a future population by a few original sur-

vivors. A similar scenario occurred less than four decades ago in the Outback of Australia.

In October of 1950, myxomatosis, caused by a virus that attacks only rabbits, was introduced into Australia to control a rabbit population of almost 600 million. The initial success was astonishing, with over 550 million animals killed. But by 1986 the rabbit population was back to over 300 million and growing. The biologists explained the failure as "a coevolution between virus and rabbits . . . [so that either] a less virulent strain of virus evolved, [or] the survivors became more resistant." Although the introduction of myxomatosis can still kill Australian rabbits, the overall death rate in the previously exposed population is now less than 30 percent.

It did not come as a surprise when immunologists found that green monkeys, like humans, have CD4 receptors on their T lymphocytes or that humans brain cells and the cells of the small and large intestine also have CD4 receptors as part of their cell walls.

The discovery of the presence of CD4 receptor sites on the surfaces of human brain cells explained for the first time the confusion, loss of short-term memory, and inability to concentrate that ultimately occur in all AIDS patients. It appears that the AIDS virus will attach itself to and infect any cell with a CD4 receptor on its surface. The CD4 receptors on cells of the stomach and in the small intestines explain the diarrhea and weight loss that is again a part of the disease. But the disease hammers away at its victims because of the CD4 receptors on the T lymphocytes themselves. We need our lymphocytes to survive. Any decrease in our T-cell population and we are left unguarded, vulnerable to attack from any bacterium, protozoa, fungus, or virus. Without our T-lymphocytes we are doomed.

In reality, it has turned out that with AIDS there is no latency period. Physicians discovered that despite some patients appearing to be in good health for years after infection, there is a continuous, gradual, but inexorable decrease in the number of the AIDS patients' CD4 T lymphocytes, not always apparent in the circulation yet, but most certainly seen in the infected patients' lymph nodes. The amounts of viral particles in a patients' lymph nodes and in the circulation, or what retrovirologists call "the viral load," doubles every two months from the moment of infection, reaching the production of a billion new viral particles a day after as little as half a year. It is clear that AIDS is a progressive disease from the very moment of infection. Of course, what was more ominous in what to the individual affected was already an ominous disease was the discovery that during this period of apparent good health, AIDS patients are the most infectious to other people.

There are some immunologists who are convinced that the development of Kaposi's sarcoma skin cancers in AIDS patients is not so much the result of direct cellular infection with the AIDS virus but represents, rather, a decrease in functioning by a damaged immune system, whose purpose is normally to patrol the body and destroy any abnormal or precancerous lesions that may begin to grow. A damaged or absent immune system means not only an increased risk of any and all kinds of infection but of cancer. And that, of course, is precisely what happens in AIDS patients.

There is not a children's hospital anywhere in the world that does not have on its infectious disease ward at least one child infected with the AIDS virus who must be given at least 150 milligrams of morphine every hour of every day to control the terrible pain of the hundreds of small malignant tumors that have developed along his or her small and large intestines.

A few AIDS specialists have presented the view that the deterioration of the immune system is caused by the body's own neutrophils and macrophages attacking infected CD4 cells in an attempt to destroy the viral infection or at least hold it in check. In essence, this immunological theory proposes that the destruction of the body's immune system is not due solely to the virus itself but to what remains of the immune system killing off its own cells in a kind of incestuous suicide.

Two Oxford scientists, Martin Nowak and Andrew McMichael, have taken this idea one step further. They have postulated that the immune systems of infected patients force the virus itself to change and, in altering itself, adapt to the attacks of the still-healthy macrophages and lymphocytes and—like bacteria becoming resistant to antibiotics—alter its own genetic code to better survive the immune attacks, passing on its new code to future generations. Using the same computer simulations as the early complexity theorists, these scientists have shown how a viral population evolves under the pressures of an immune attack. In the model, a virus infecting T cells is clearly held in check until, in some of the hosts, a change in the genetic code of the virus reaches the genes that produce the outer protein coat. For a time the host's killer T cells are able to kill enough infected cells and the body's B cells able to make enough specific antibody to bind up any free-floating viral particles; but eventually the mutations alter the viral proteins of the outer coat. The new mutant viruses are able to multiply and divide, setting up the immune collapse that eventually leads to full-blown clinical AIDS. Such mutational changes do appear to be happening. In Thailand a new strain of the AIDS virus, more adapted to heterosexual spread, is becoming the dominant virus in the spread of the disease.

After a decade of infection, it is crystal clear to everyone that the AIDS virus, unlike other viruses willing to cut a kind of parasitic deal with their host to live and let live, has no interest in anything other than infecting a cell, killing it, and moving on.

25

The future is not what it used to be.

PAUL VALÉRY

All science, like any human enterprise, is ultimately a story. There are villains and heroes, fools and charlatans, successes and failures. The story changes with the circumstances, while the major themes of one age become the discarded myths of the next.

The successes and myths of medicine, the most human of all sciences, are a bit easier to follow than those of physics or mathematics because medicine, with its theories and their practical applications, so intimately affects each of us, becoming personal and, as we become ill, immediate. For most of human history the stories remained much the same . . . disturbed humors, the intervention of the stars, imbalances of hot and cold, poisons and vapors, curses and sins, good pus and bad pus. It has only been in the last 150 years that the century-old stories have been replaced, first by careful observation and then by science itself.

There have been three great advances in this new era of scientific medicine. The first was sanitation, spurred on by Pasteur's germ theory of disease; the second was the discovery of anesthesia, giving surgeons the ability to perform both prolonged and intricate procedures; and third, most recently—indeed less than fifty years ago—was the advance that has established the present view of disease, indeed of all illness: specifically the discovery of antibiotics and the ability to treat and cure infections.

The whole notion of stopping disease, not to mention curing it, was simply unthought of before the discovery of penicillin. The idea of the "magic bullet" has now become so powerful and so pervasive that today cardiovascular surgeons talk about stopping heart disease, while rheumatologists, though well aware that they are dealing with a chronic degenerative condition, play to an expectant and demanding audience with announcements of better and more effective nonsteroidal anti-inflammatory drugs and new curative treatments. The infectious disease story of Pasteur, Koch, Lister, Jenner, Fleming, and Salk has displaced all the other narratives and, in the process, become its own myth.

But no story is ever complete, every narrative eventually loses its audience, and under the pressures of conflict and change, it may ultimately lose its relevance. In a society in which an aging population makes chronic emphysema, degenerative joint disease, prostate cancer, and strokes the defining problems; in which coronary artery bypasses inevitably clog up again; in which bacteria grow resistant and malaria and tuberculosis again strike down the poor and the helpless; and where the new viral infections become lifelong affairs, the magic-bullet model no longer fits and a once-useful narrative is not only useless but becomes a dangerous illusion.

There just is no surgical procedure or antibiotic to cure a sixty-five-year-old with emphysema or severe erosive rheumatoid arthritis; no treatment for an 840-gram infant with class four intracerebral bleeding; no penicillin left to treat a methicillin-resistant staphyloccal infection; and no real hope for a vaccine against AIDS.

But there is certainly an enormous effort, if not to cure AIDS, at least to treat the infection, to do what physicians have always tried to do and what has always given medicine its value: to relieve suffering and treat the treatable.

In theory, the treatment of AIDS should be simple, but in practice it has proven quite difficult. The problem is that with the retroviruses we must reverse 3.5 billion years of evolution and find ways to stop the attachment of the virus to susceptible cells, inhibit the action of reverse transcriptase, interfere with the assembly enzymes and the nucleases that cut cellular DNA to insert a copy of viral genes. It is no easy task and so far we have not been very effective.

It is a new world, with new dangers and new victims. Nowhere is the new story more clearly seen than with the retroviruses, already the major cause of death in young adults between the ages of eighteen and thirty-five and the major cause of mental retardation in newborns. But there are other new stories. Edward Golub, in his book *The Limits of Medicine*, may have been more prophetic than even he would have wished:

> In this half century we have learned to think about disease and dying as unnatural, as enemies to be fought and vanquished. We don't talk about people dying from cancer or other chronic diseases, we talk about their losing the battle; scientists do work to find causes and cures, they battle deadly bacillus; physicians do battle with disease and death. Infectious diseases lent themselves to the imagery—microbes *do* invade; and the body does respond—but the metaphor has failed us with chronic, degenerative, and genetic diseases.

Nowhere is the need for a new metaphor clearer than in the spread to humans of mad cow disease. Here is a story not only with an unexpected ending but, like so much of biology, a story that appears to have begun at the very beginnings of evolution.

There would seem to be no connection between a strange occurrence in the genetics of yeast and the transmission of a degenerative brain disease. But there is a terrible arrogance in assuming that there is nothing new and that we are all not connected to everything else.

Early in the study of inheritance, biologists turned to yeast as a preferred organism for experimentation. Yeasts have a small number of genes, have rapid generation times, and are easily grown in large numbers. It was soon discovered that the different colors of yeast were transmitted to future generations in a reproducible and clearly inherited manner. But the molecular geneticists could find no differences in the sequences of nucleotides in the different-colored organisms, yet brown yeast still gave rise to brown yeasts and gray yeasts to gray yeasts. Reluctantly the researchers came to the conclusion that the transmission of color was an even earlier form of heredity, a method of passing on physical characteristics to future generations that had nothing to do with nucleotides, replicating polymers, or DNA. The scientists thought that this inheritance had something to do with the transmission of proteins, a remnant of a prebiological form of heredity that preceded the evolution of nucleic acids that had been retained in this earliest form of cellular life. The question that wasn't asked was whether this type of hereditary protein transfer might be maintained in the higher animals.

In the early 1980s the methods for rendering animal carcasses in England were changed and the change became more than academic. The changes for rendering dead animals were made for purely economic reasons. Temperatures at rendering plants were decreased from 187 degrees to 160 degrees Fahrenheit, saving fuel costs, while surveillance of animals in regard to previous diseases was reduced. Needing a cheap supplement to maintain increased milk production on English farms having little acreage for grazing, the English dairy industry added the viscera and trimmings of butchered sheep and goats as well as once-discarded bone meal to the commercial animal feeds as a caloric supplement. Scrapie, a degenerative and universally fatal neurological disease of sheep and goats, named for the fact that these diseased animals develop such an intense itch that they scrape off their fur or wool, was present in some English herds whose animals were used for these food supplements. There were veterinarians who warned that these changes in processing might lead to contamination, since it was assumed that scrapie was caused by a virus. Indeed, diseases similar to scrapie had been found to be present in mink, mule deer, elk, and cows. In cows it was given the name bovine spongiform encephalopathy because of the holes found in the brains of these animals at autopsy. But the British agricultural industry and governmental agencies silenced the critics by stating that heating the supplements to temperatures of 160 degrees would destroy any bacteria as well as any known viruses.

Similar degenerative diseases were also found to occur in humans under the exotic names of kuru, Gerstmann-Sträussler-Scheinker disease, fatal insomnia, and Creutzfeldt-Jakob disease. Kuru was a disease restricted to the inhabitants of New Guinea, where a detailed epidemiological analysis proved that the disease was passed from person to person through the practice of ritual cannibalism. The practice was stopped in the late 1950s and by the late 1980s the disease was no longer present on the island. Creutzfeldt-Jakob, in contrast to kuru, is a worldwide disease with an incidence of one per million. Some cases of the disease appear to be inherited, but by the late 1970s it was clear that, like kuru, it could be spread through inadvertent cross contamination. The detective work done by neurologists using Snow's statistical approach showed that the disease was transmitted from patients with the disease, or from those who would later develop the condition, through exposure to diseased brains during neurological operative procedures as well as strange dietary customs such as occurred in a group of Libyan Jews who consumed lightly cooked sheep brains and eyeballs as a delicacy. What was distressing to these neurologists was that the disease was clearly transmitted between patients and, in some cases, to the neurosurgeons operating on the brains of these patients, presumably through inadvertent punctures, using surgical instruments that had been properly sterilized. It was Semmelweis all over again, only this time the instruments had been sterilized. The implications were obvious. If this disease was caused by a virus, it was a virus impervious to heat—and worse, the studies indicated an enormously long incubation period. The average age of onset of the disease in human populations was in the middle sixties.

A theory had been presented by virologists that these neurological diseases were due to a new species of a "slow virus," a virus that infected cells early in the individual's life only to cause neurological degeneration and death decades later. This slow virus concept ignored the surgical instrument data, but science does constantly reform itself, and any time there is a disease with no explanation, viruses are always invoked.

And that was precisely the situation with regard to the degenerative neurological diseases until the 1980s when the incidence of mad cow disease in England began to escalate, striking down hundreds and then thousands of British cows. The milk and beef industry asked the scientists for help. It was quickly discovered that the disease could be transmitted from sick animals to healthy ones by the injection of extracts from the brains of diseased animals into the central nervous system of healthy controls. The veterinarians at the Central Veterinary Laboratory in Weybridge traced the source of the emerging epidemic to the new food supplements that contained meat and bone meal of dead sheep. They discovered that the disease could be caused by eating the contaminated feed or by simple exposure to it and that direct injection of diseased tissue was not necessary.

There was no doubt that mad cow disease was caused by a transmissible infectious agent, but no one could find a virus—a fast or a slow one. Electron micrographs of diseased brains never revealed a single viral particle; more surprising was the fact that exposure of diseased brain extracts to large doses of ultraviolet ionizing radiation as well as mixtures of toxic chemicals at levels known to destroy any and all DNA or RNA still left the extracts infectious. One of the old stories of science is that DNA and RNA are the operational foundations of life. The fact that study after study showed the absence of any sequences of viral nucleotides in any of the obviously infectious material stood modern science on its head. Molecular studies of the infectious material did show the presence of a small protein not present in the brains of normal animals. It was all terribly confusing until a few researchers, relying on what they'd observed, decided to ignore both authority and dogma and proposed that the transmissible agent was not a virus or any substance that contained DNA or RNA, transfer nucleotides, or nucleases but special proteins that they called "prions," for *proteinaceous infectious particles.* It was both a new and old story. These researchers concluded that prions could be transmitted from cell to cell and, like all proteins, were incredibly resistant to both heat and acids. It was proposed that prions cause disease not by taking over the genetic codes of a cell but by actually binding to normal cytoplasmic proteins and causing them to change their three-dimensional shapes into shapes that produce cellular dysfunction.

Today an enormous amount of new information has proven these scientists to be correct. Prions are responsible for a number of inheritable disorders and, at least in yeasts, for the transmission of the characteristics of color. Prions may very well be an additional means of inheritance in humans as well as a cause for disease.

In short, a new kind of infectious disease had been discovered. Neurologists at Hammersmith Hospital in London warned the British government about the potential dangers of their animal food supplements and the possibility of cross contamination to humans but were dismissed.

In 1990 the neurologists, ignoring the British government's

pronouncement of safety, set up their own epidemiological surveillance program to monitor the incidence of Creutzfeldt-Jakob disease in humans. The idea was quite simple; there was an epidemic of an infectious disease in cows that was known to be transferable across species lines. It was also known that the agent causing the disease could be spread by simple contact or ingestion and that the agent was resistant to destruction by the normal means of heating.

In April of 1996 *The Lancet* published an article entitled, "A New Variant of Creutzfeldt-Jakob Disease in the United Kingdom." The article documented the history and course of ten patients. The ages at the death of these patients ranged from nineteen to forty-one years. The interval between the onset of their neurological disease, beginning with episodes of poor coordination, progressing to seizures and ultimately death, was a very short 3.5 to 22.5 months. Examination at autopsy of these patients' brains showed lesions similar to those described in scrapie and mad cow disease. One of those who died had worked as a butcher; another had visited an abattoir for two days in 1987; another had spent a week's holiday on a dairy farm in the late 1980s. All the patients had reported to have eaten beef or beef products but not brains.

The Lancet article ended its report, "Exposure of the human population to the bovine spongiform encephalopathy agent is likely to have been greatest in the 1980s. This is consistent with an incubation period of between five and ten years. Additional studies released by the U. K. Ministry of Agriculture, Fisheries, and Food indicate that mad cow disease can be passed vertically from cow to calf. This type of maternal transmission was already known to occur in scrapie. Despite these new studies, the British government advisory committee has stated 'There is no case for changing its recommendations in relationship to milk, meat, blood, or other products.'"

It is now feared that the human contamination in England

may be widespread, and if this is indeed true, hundreds of additional cases of the variant of Creutzfeldt-Jakob disease will appear over the next decade, while presumably the British government and its cattle and milk industry will continue debating whether they should slaughter some or all of their 14 million cows.

If the stories of AIDS, mad cow disease, and Creutzfeldt-Jakob disease are cautionary tales, they are also the vanguard of a whole new set of biological stories in which the old methods of containment, treatment, and cures no longer work.

Agricultural corporations are today inserting genes into plants to increase the plant's insect resistance, add more sugar content to its juices, or provide for longer shelf life. The corporations insist that the spread of these inserted genes outside of their plants is not an issue. But recently these corporations received two rude shocks from the scientific community. The first was the observation that an engineered Brazil-nut gene placed in soybeans intended for animal feed to provide additional protein content caused severe allergic reactions when the genetically altered soybeans were tested on people. The second and more alarming discovery was the observation that a gene inserted into seed grains to make the plants resistant to certain herbicides, offering the promise of a wheat crop that will not be harmed by the proper use of herbicides, has made its way into the wild grasses surrounding the test plots. It is clear that there still is a great deal to learn about the submicroscopic world of evolution and a great deal of mystery left to unravel in how genes work, how they move around nature, as well as exactly how they function. It was only recently that retrovirologists studying the life cycle of the AIDS virus showed that during infection the viral genes induce the cellular production of a specific protein that enhances the transcription of normal cellular genes, increasing the ability of the infected cell to proliferate. In short, not only does the AIDS virus take over cellular machinery to make more viruses, but during its own evolution it developed proteins that stimulate an infected cell to increase its cellular proliferation in order to increase the numbers of cells carrying forward the virus's own genes, ensuring the virus a better chance for its own survival.

It is now thought that an AIDS virus, once inside a CD4 cell, actually activates cellular genes that downregulate cellular surface markers, specifically the class I markers, making the infected cell invisible to the body's surviving immune system. The infected cells then become the stealth bombers of the infection, carrying the virus into uninfected areas undetected by what remains of the patient's already damaged immune system. But what nature takes away, it can also give. There have always been those few people exposed to the AIDS virus who do not develop the disease. The African physicians have followed a few dozen prostitutes in Uganda who have been constantly exposed to the virus but have never developed full blown AIDS; in this country and in Europe there are those one or two who, despite injections with contaminated needles, remain healthy. The question has always been why, and after a decade of study the answer is clear . . . it is the green monkey story all over again.

The AIDS virus needs a CD4 receptor site to begin its invasion of human cells, but this coupling also needs the participation of an additional, smaller membrane receptor. Patients who are resistant to HIV infection have a mutation in the gene that codes for that coreceptor. Genetic diversity has produced a very small subset of humans whose cells, because of this mutation, are resistant to infection with the AIDS virus. In short, no matter how great or widespread the epidemic, there will be those few in Africa and India, in New York and Paris who will survive and pass on the mutated gene to future generations so that if nothing is done, after a few thousand years, the descendants of these few survivors will repopulate the earth and AIDS will be no more than another mild flulike illness. But now, for most of us, as for the green monkeys of a half million years ago, the world has changed and there will be no going back.

26

Life is short, the art long, opportunity fleeting, experience treacherous, judgment difficult. The physician must be ready, not only to do his duty himself, but also to secure the cooperation of the patient, of the attendants, and of the eternals.

HIPPOCRATES (460–375 B.C.)

At the end of the first millennium, a second sun suddenly appeared in the heavens. The new sun burned brightly throughout the day and night, throwing the world into social chaos. From Constantinople to the Nile epidemics were blamed on the appearance of this new star. The Chinese and Arabic literature set the date of the sun's appearance at July 4th of the year 1054. The new sun burned for twenty-three days, and then as quickly as it had appeared, it vanished. At a time when Galenic teaching dominated European medicine, defining melancholia as a result of too much black bile and all health and disease as imbalances of food and drink, sleep and waking, evacuation and repletion, motion and rest, passion and emotion, the presence of this second sun cast into doubt the accepted therapeutic doctrine of balances, unsettling the whole system of rules and judgments based as they were on the assumptions of celestial perfection. Almost a thousand years after the second sun's appearance, the remnant of the supernova, now a neutron star, was discovered spinning in the center of the Crab nebula.

The first millennium of human history ended with an all-too-human occurrence, the interposition of a misinterpreted physical event into the issues of health and disease; and for another 800 years, except for the efforts of a few courageous scientists, very little changed. Doctors and surgeons continued to treat and prescribe on the basis of sectarian dogmas or mere speculation; political authorities took little responsibility for the removal of contagion, while religious authorities caught up in the midst of disease and death confessed the penitent and prayed for divine mercy. But just as we reach the end of this millennium having finally discovered the explanation for that second sun whose presence closed out the first, we also end the millennium with a realistic understanding of disease, a glimpse of the new stories that are beginning to unfold, and the hard-won knowledge of what we must do to keep ourselves and our children alive. It is how we handle this information that will set the tone for the next millennium.

At a 1986 international meeting of retrovirologists, Gallo and Montagnier, in the spirit of conciliation, agreed to name the AIDS virus *HIV*, for human immune deficiency virus. It is the name that will be used until the end of human history.

The first article to use this new designation did not mince words: "The [HIV] produced by cultured T cells from patients with AIDS and pre-AIDS is highly infectious and can be readily transmitted to adult peripheral blood and bone marrow lymphocytes."

But while the lethality of the virus was becoming more and more obvious, so were other crucial observations. The first was that the virus was not transmitted through the air; nor did it hide on toilet seats or lurk in dusty closets; it was not in the water or food supply; it did not exist in sweat; mosquitos could not transmit it; nor was it carried from place to place on people's hands.

The virus exists only in human serums and CD4 cells and can only be transmitted through exposure to already-infected blood, serums, tissues, or organs. AIDS has been reported in patients who have received transplanted organs from HIV-positive donors, and in June of 1996 *The Lancet* reported the first documented transmission of HIV by a human bite.

But above all, it is the overwhelming lethality of this infection that so concerns anyone who becomes HIV-positive, cares for AIDS patients, does AIDS research, or looks for an AIDS vaccine. The plain and simple fact is that at the present time virtually no one in Africa, Europe, North America, India, Asia, or anywhere else in the world is alive eight years after their circulating CD4 T lymphocytes begin to fall below 100 cells per cubic millimeter of blood.

Unlike the early 1980s, the epidemic is now so devastating and widespread that countries no longer feel the need to suppress medical data. In Kenya 15 percent of pregnant women are now HIV-positive; in Kanazulu, South Africa, the figure is 8 percent; in Francistown, Botswana, 34 percent of pregnant women are HIV-positive, a rate that has quadrupled between 1991 and 1993. It is the adolescents, specifically adolescent girls, who are now falling prey to the HIV virus and passing the virus onto their newborns. The heartland of Africa is facing a bleak and terrible future.

Asia, with its 4 billion people, is currently experiencing the most rapidly growing epidemic of AIDS in the world. Since 1992 the numbers of Asians infected with HIV has doubled to over a million.

In 1995 the first reported incidence of the heterosexual Thailand strain of HIV was reported in three airmen stationed at the Travis Air Force base in California. The medieval distinctions of high-risk and low-risk groups that so many have hidden behind and that politicians have so righteously exploited are gone. At the eighth annual meeting of the National Cooperative Vaccine Development Groups for AIDS held in 1995 at Bethesda, Maryland, researchers from England reported that HIV type E, the viral subtype more easily spread through vaginal intercourse than HIV-1, the present major subtype infecting the U.S. population, has already overtaken HIV-1 as the major virus in Thailand and certain other parts of Asia and India.

Inexplicably, there is still no public outcry. Yet business communities around the world find that they are no longer able to ignore the effect of AIDS on their work force, markets, and lending policies. Business executives of worldwide conglomerates are finally seeing the risks the virus brings to their own enterprises in the increasing incidence of AIDS in truckers in Indiana and miners in South Africa and are beginning to devise their own prevention programs. It would certainly have been better if indeed AIDS acted like cholera or puerperal fever, if there were vomiting and diarrhea, suffering and death within hours of infection. Then governments and public health agencies would have been forced to do anything or everything. But the long incubation period and the protracted, lingering deaths that have allowed AIDS patients to be sequestered in hospices or upstairs bedrooms of friends and relatives have permitted physicians to waffle, public health officials to make political statements, and politicians to show cold indifference.

A recent study on sexual activity of high school students shows that over 40 percent are sexually active before graduation, yet none think about AIDS, while a new generation of homosexuals refuses to practice safe sex, and drug users continue to share contaminated needles. Biology, whether in the Cambrian age, Iowa, or San Francisco, can be ignored but never avoided. Retroviruses, too, have their own schemes and their own methods. The world can run but it can't hide. The spread of the virus in the late 1980s through Brazil was along the old heroin routes.

The answers to the new stories will have less to do with new tests and new treatments than they will with sympathy, understanding, and prevention. The fact that anticipation, prevention, and concern will have to become the new solutions of medicine is not so surprising; they are the very qualities that have always given medicine its true value and its real power to both comfort and heal.

In Holland the incidence of AIDS has decreased 30 percent with the distribution of free needles to drug abusers. It is a biological fact that the tiny blood transfusions that occur when intravenous drug users share needles is the single most efficient way to transmit the AIDS virus from person to person—decidedly more efficient than sexual activity, homosexual or heterosexual. It is also a fact that once the HIV virus is established in a drug culture, it moves out into the surrounding society through sexual contact and pregnancy. It is also a fact that one-third of all new AIDS cases in the United States can be traced back in some way to the injection of an illicit substance and that drug users are now the main reservoirs of the disease in the cities of North America and Europe.

Yet, in the United States, prescriptions are required to purchase injection products such as needles and syringes. It is also illegal for people to possess equipment for administering drugs, even if they don't purchase syringes. As a national policy, the purchase of clean needles is a criminal offense.

Unfortunately, this kind of official craziness is part of the whole issue of condoms. It has been proven that modern latex condoms *do* work to stop the spread of sexually transmitted AIDS, despite the archaic and flawed studies from the early 1960s with nonlatex condoms that today's condom opponents, with the supportive silence of our politicans, dredge up to show that only abstinence works. Modern condoms, if used properly, do not break and do not allow the passage of the AIDS virus and offer 100 percent protection for a 100 percent fatal and always brutal disease; not bad odds when it is also a fact that today in the United States 1 in 200 of what are euphemistically called non–high-risk individuals are nevertheless infected with the virus and don't even know they are infected and don't look as if they are HIV-positive.

But just as Snow's detractors ridiculed and disparaged his maps, today those whose propaganda and strident views use AIDS to promote their own causes and push their own agendas once again ignore the statistics and the science, putting their own families and indeed all of us at risk. In truth, we know beyond a reasonable doubt that AIDS is as much a disease of how we live as it is a disease of retroviral replication. It is a disease with which, if we are to save ourselves, we simply have to care about everyone else.

The irony of AIDS is that for the first time in human history a disease that is fatal is totally preventable without the need for isolation or quarantine, immunization, injections, a dozen pills a day, or vaccinations. One would assume that at the very least the medical community would be insisting on programs and public health measures be put into place and that we use all we already know to stop the spread of this disease.

It may be one of the greatest secrets in medicine, but AIDS prevention programs are successful, but the successes are a direct function of when and where those programs are implemented. Specifically, prevention programs are successful where prevalence of AIDS among drug users is low and where the spread into the homosexual population is not yet extensive. Community drug outreach programs, access to sterile injection equipment, and over-the-counter pharmacy sales of injection equipment have kept rates of HIV conversions low compared to communities without such programs, and in some areas today these measures are even leading to declining rates of HIV spread among drug addicts.

The worldwide AIDS studies by John K. Walters of the Uni-

versity of California, Kachet Chomupanga of the Bangkok Met-
ropolitan Administration, Rueland A. Coutinho of the Munici-
pal Health Service of Amsterdam, and Afredo Nicolusi of the
National Research Council in Milan have all shown similar results. It is a fact that where drug treatment programs reduce ad-
diction and where individuals can be kept from injecting drugs,
the number of AIDS cases is reduced even in areas where sero-
prevalence is high. But when all this is ignored and data are
scorned, when children continue to be born infected, college students become HIV-positive, and physicians and nurses continue
to stick their fingers when drawing blood, everyone has to wonder if it is not all of us who have gone crazy.

In 1862, writer and philosopher Samuel Butler set the record
straight not only for his age, but for ours: "Let us settle the facts
first and fight about the moral tendencies later."

Yet in 1995, Congress passed Public Law 102–394, which
clearly stated, ". . . no funds appropriated under this act shall be
used to carry out any program of distributing sterile needles for
the hypodermic injection of any illicit drug. . . ." In an elegantly
controlled study from Baltimore, diabetic patients who were
also drug abusers, using clean syringes and needles, had an HIV-
infection rate less than half that of the nondiabetic drug users.

In Africa the spread of HIV is mainly through heterosexual
transmission. But the African physicians are learning. Education
and simple treatments have decreased the transmission rate
from over 35 percent to below 24 percent in sexually active
Ugandan women. However, the African men, at best, remain
cavalier about the spread of the disease and, at worst, simply
refuse to be concerned about their HIV status. There are wom-
en's groups in Africa that are convinced women must simply
learn to protect themselves, that it is women who must be em-
powered, demand condom use, petition the politicians, argue
with their ministers, not only to save themselves, but their chil-

dren. By refusing to discuss how to stay alive, we are dooming ourselves to die.

It is no secret that bacteria and viruses have always taken advantage of any and all opportunities. In the past the most vulnerable have been the very young and the elderly, those whose immunity has not yet developed or those whose immune systems are in decline; but today infectious diseases are spreading fastest among young adults. It is this group now who share contaminated needles, have unprotected sex, or live together in crowded apartments who have become the most vulnerable.

But the increase in the incidence of both viral and bacterial infections is greatest in young women, and certainly in young pregnant women. Women have never been a priority in a male-dominated medical establishment. They have been excluded from scientific studies, ignored in regard to new treatments, and misdiagosed in regard to illnesses. The truth is that men and women are different and have different responses and different susceptibility to infections. The whole process of conception presents a woman with a different set of general medical problems and specific biological issues. Increases in circulating estrogens rev up the immune system. Molecules of the hormone estrogen increase activity of the T and B cells that lie in the uterus. In a very real way the lining of the uterus is open to the outside world, and it benefits a woman to have a more effective immune system patrolling her uterus to attack and destroy any wandering bacteria or viruses gaining entrance to the uterus through the vagina. But this increased activity also leads to an increased incidence of the autoimmune diseases. During pregnancy, a woman not only has to carry a developing fetus but she must protect the embryo's cells with their different surface markers from an immune system that, if given the chance, would attack and certainly destroy them.

In fact, during pregnancy estrogen levels drop off and a woman's immune system is downgraded; the immunity of the uterus, fallopian tubes, and cervix is diminished so that the fetus is not attacked, but this allows for increased bacterial and viral survival and growth. The T and B cells of pregnant women can no longer clearly distinguish self from nonself cells, which makes every pregnant women more susceptible to the spread of disease.

The rules of infection are simply not the same for men and for women, any more than the rules of the retroviral infection are the same as the rules for DNA viruses or that mad cow disease is the same as anthrax.

This disconnect between what we know and how we act became excruciatingly clear in a miniepidemic of *Haemophilus influenzae* meningitis in Mankato, Minnesota. The epidemic brought out the full resources of the state and federal governments. Ten thousand people were immunized with the *H. influenzae* vaccine; another 5,000 were given the antibiotic rifampin to eliminate those that might be carriers of the organism. Schools and shopping malls were closed. One father interviewed on television ignored the obvious inconvenience and enormous cost explaining, "With such a dangerous disease, everything has to be done no matter what the cost or inconvenience." Apparently the state and federal governments, the board of health, politicians, town physicians, teachers, school superintendents, mall owners, and the majority of the Mankato community felt the same. Some parents even condemned the public meetings that had been held to explain the disease, believing the meetings might themselves be a means of spreading the bacteria. Yet, it is fair to state that at a time when only six students developed meningitis, no one in Mankato was aware that during that same week the Centers for Disease Control in Atlanta released a report stating that AIDS had become the leading cause of death in people between the ages of eighteen and forty-five, far exceeding accidents, homicides, or cancer, and that for the preceeding five years over 20 percent of all new AIDS cases occurred in the twenty-to-twenty-nine-year-old age range, adults clearly infected while in grammar and high school while still in their teens and preteens. Indeed, the majority of people in Mankato had opposed AIDS and sex education in their public schools, ignoring the obvious, that one out of five adolescents in America contracts a sexually transmitted disease and that 70 percent of all twelfth-graders are sexually active. In the world or in the Mankatos of America, death, almost in secret, haunts what was once the healthiest segment of the community.

But humans are not stupid and we are not without great resources. We still have our Harveys and Semmelweises, our Pasteurs, Gallos and our Hos. The truth is that the AIDS scenario has happened before. We have all made this particular fight before, and we won that battle with considerably fewer resources and a great deal less knowledge than is available today.

Syphilis, like AIDS, was once the unspoken disease, a sexually transmitted infection with a long incubation period resulting ultimately in heart failure, congenital malformations, blindness, dementia, mental retardation, psychosis, and death. Uncles and aunts died in secret, hidden away from friends and relatives. Politicians and ministers spoke out against immorality, while since the discovery of penicillin thousands of times a year physicians were forced to conjure up fictitious conditions in order to give two weeks of intramuscular antibiotic injections to the exposed wives and mistresses of infected husbands and lovers, hoping that any infants would not be born with the blindness and heart disease of congenital syphilis.

During the 1930s and 1940s, syphilis had become endemic in China. By 1948 it was estimated that fully 40 percent of the population of China's major cities was infected; yet in less than three decades the disease was eliminated from Shanghai, Canton, and Peking, and from all of the towns of its major provinces as surely as Jenner had eliminated smallpox and Jonas Salk banished polio.

In 1949 the new Chinese government was overwhelmed and understood that nothing could be accomplished, from industrialization to land reform, with so large a part of the population ill. Clearly fearing a social meltdown, it enlisted the help of the world's experts on syphilis, organized its medical establishment as well as the population, and made the elimination of syphilis from China as much a political objective as a public health goal. Despite the disease's transmission being sexual, with all the accompanying social and cultural prejudices, the government persevered attacking the epidemic as a medical problem and an issue of individual responsibility.

There are a number of historians who consider the eradication of syphilis from a population of a half billion people in less than thirty years to be the single greatest public health success in all of human history. What is certain is that the epidemic was eliminated by a conviction on the part of both government and medicine to save its people.

This millennium will end and we will start the next with a population of over 6 billion people and a human growth rate of another 10 million a year. The census of the major cities of the world, Bombay, Mexico City, New York, and Bangkok will have increased by 30 percent in the next five years. Our science is not being stretched, we are. Medicine can handle our problems. It can do what good medicine has always done, what has given it value and honor in every generation. It can explain connections, how we live and how we die; be an advocate for the ill and the suffering; serve the individual and support the weak. The answer for the next thousand years is the same as that for the last thousand. It is the answer of Paracelsus, of Jenner, Gallo, and Snow, "Go back to the bedside, back to observation and experiment, to look . . . to be suspicious of eloquence, ignore ceremony, lecture and write in the common language, proceed from reason, and move on the learning of experience."

The world has always been a ruthless place. It has always

been dangerous out there. In the long struggle for existence, survival has never been assured to anyone or granted to anything. It has always had to be fought for and pursued . . . but winning now is the same as winning then, a continuation of the past and the knowledge that there will always be a future.

THE END

Citations / Recommended Readings

Chapter 1

Graham, John R. "*Helicobacter pylori*: Human Pathogen or Simply an Opportunist." *Lancet* 345 (1995): 1095–1096.

Monmany, Terence. "Annals of Medicine, Marshall's Hunch." *New Yorker* (20 September 1993): 64–72.

Shallcross, T.M., Tompkins, D.S., Rathbone, B.J. "Mucosal IgA Recognition of *Helicobacter pylori* 120 KDa Protein, Peptic Ulceration, and Gastric Pathology." *Lancet* 338 (1991): 332–335.

Chapter 4

Rebek, J., Jr. "Molecular Recognition and Self-Replication" [Review]. *Journal of Molecular Recognition* 5(3) (1992): 83–88.

Chapter 9

Brunet, J.B. "Acquired Immunodeficiency Syndrome in France." *Lancet* (26 March 1983): 700–701.

Waldrop, M. Mitchell. *Complexity, The Emerging Science at the Edge of Order and Chaos.* New York: Simon & Shuster, 1992.

Watson, James D. *The Double Helix.* New York: Atheneum, 1968.

Chapter 13

Dubos, René. *Louis Pasteur, Freelance of Science.* New York: Charles Scribner's Sons, 1950, 1976.

Gleick, James. *Genius, The Life and Science of Richard Feynman.* New York: Pantheon Books, 1992.

Gore, Rick, Mazzatenta, O. Louis. "The Cambrian Period Explosion of Life." *National Geographic* (October 1993): 120–136.

Young, Jeffrey. "Lefties, Righties and Anxieties." *Forbes* (19 July 1993): 208.

Chapter 14

"Update on Acquired Immune Deficiency Syndrome (AIDS)—United States." *Morbidity and Mortality Weekly Report* 31(37) (1982): 507–508, 513–514.

Gagnon, John H., et al. *Sex in America*. Boston: Little Brown & Company, 1994.

Chapter 16

Puchin, Jeffrey S., et al. "Hantavirus Pulmonary Syndrome: A Clinical Description of Seventeen Patients With a Newly Recognized Disease." *New England Journal of Medicine* 330 (1994): 949–955.

Seale, J. "Crossing the Species Barrier—Viruses and the Origins of AIDS in Perspective" [Review]. *Journal of the Royal Society of Medicine* 82(9) (1989): 519–523.

Chapter 18

Parkman, Robertson, Weinberg, Kenneth. "Age, The Thymus and T Lymphocytes." *New England Journal of Medicine* 332 (1995): 182–183.

Chapter 19

Shilts, Randy. *And The Band Played On: Politics, People and the AIDS Epidemic*. New York: St. Martins Press, 1987.

Chapter 20

Cleary, Michael L. A "Promiscuous Oncogene in Acute Leukemia." *New England Journal of Medicine* 329: 958–959.

Huebner, R.J., Todara, G.J. "Oncogenes of RNA Tumor Viruses as Determinants of Cancer." *Proceedings of the National Academy of Sciences of the United States of America* 64 (1969): 1087–1094.

Huebner, R.J., Todara, G.J. "N.A.S. Symposium: New Evidence as the Basis for Increased Efforts in Cancer Research" [Review]. *Proceedings of the National Academy of Sciences of the United States of America* 69 (1972): 1009–1015.

Chapter 21
Case Records of the Massachusetts General Hospital. *New England Journal of Medicine* 333: 1485–1493.

Chapter 23
Barre-Sinoussi, F., et al. "Isolation of a T-Lymphocyte Retrovirus from a Patient at Risk for Acquired Immune Deficiency Syndrome." *Science* 220 (1983): 868–870.
Gallo, R.C., et al. "Human T-Cell Leukemia-Lymphoma Virus (HTLV) Is in T- but not B-Lymphocytes from a Patient with Cutaneous T-Cell Lymphomas." *Proceedings of the National Academy of Sciences of the United States of America* 79 (1982): 5680–5683.

Chapter 24
Seife, Charles. "The Harebrained Scheme." *Scientific American* (February 1996): 24–26.

Chapter 25
Gajdusek, D.C. "Unconventional Viruses and the Origins and Disappearance of Kuru." *Science* 197 (1977): 943–960.
Golub, Edward S. *The Limits of Medicine.* New York: Random House, Times Books, 1994.
Prusiner, Stanley B. "The Prior Disease." *Scientific American* (January 1995).
Will, R.G., et al. "A New Variant of Creutzfeldt-Jakob Disease in the United Kingdom." *Lancet* 347 (1996): 921–925.

Chapter 26
Brecher, Kenneth. "A Near-Eastern Sighting of the Super Nova Explosion of 1054." *Nature* 273 (1978): 728–730.
Choopanya, K., et al. "International Epidemiology of HIV and AIDS Among Injecting Drug Users." *AIDS* 10 (1992): 1053–1068.
Coming Clean About Needle Exchange. *Lancet* 346 (1995): 1377.
Des Jarlais, Don C., Friedman, Samuel R. "AIDS and the Use of Injected Drugs." *Scientfic American* (February 1994).
Kimball, Ann Marie, Thant, Myo. "A Role for Business in HIV Prevention in Asia." *Lancet* 347 (1996): 70–72.